The Yellow Demon of Fever

The Yellow Demon of Fever

Fighting Disease in the Nineteenth-Century Transatlantic Slave Trade

Manuel Barcia

Yale

UNIVERSITY PRESS

New Haven & London

Published with assistance from the foundation established in memory of Philip Hamilton
McMillan of the Class of 1894, Yale College.

Yale University Press books may be purchased in quantity for educational, business, or
promotional use. For information, please e-mail sales.press@yale.edu (U.S. office) or
sales@yaleup.co.uk (U.K. office).

Set in Bulmer by IDS Infotech, Ltd.
Printed in the United States of America.

Library of Congress Control Number: 2019940122
ISBN 978-0-300-21585-4 (hardcover : alk. paper)

A catalogue record for this book is available from the British Library.

This paper meets the requirements of ANSI/NISO Z39.48-1992 (Permanence of Paper).

10 9 8 7 6 5 4 3 2 1

For Effie and Kenny

Insular America has not been much rummaged by professional travellers. The yellow demon of fever, with huge red eyes, glares so terrifically at them, that they drop their portfolios in affright.

—Robert Jameson, *Letters from the Havana*

Contents

Acknowledgments

THIS BOOK IS the result of years of research, research that originally was nothing more than taking notes about curious aspects of the medical history of the Atlantic during the so-called illegal era of the slave trade, while examining documents that concerned previous book projects. Over time, the amount of information became so overwhelming that I found myself at a crossroads, wondering whether I should go ahead and turn myself into a historian of medicine (an enterprise that is still a limping project of its own), or whether I should simply use all this information as curious snippets to inform my work focusing on other aspects of the slave trade. Ultimately, the former enterprise won and did so handsomely. I began devouring everything published on the topic, and repeatedly bothering some colleagues at the top of the field, such as Katherine Paugh and Pablo Gómez. Without their generous advice and comments, I would have run this project into the ground, even before it had taken off.

In all truth, I have been blessed with colleagues who are more often than not also wonderful friends, and who have shared information on a regular basis. I fear that I might forget someone here, but among those who have never failed me are Richard Anderson, María del Carmen Barcia, Lloyd Belton, Alex Borucki, Jorge Felipe, Rebecca Goetz, Dale Graden, John Harris, Kalle Kanooja, Henry Lovejoy, Leonardo Marques, the late Joe Miller, Jennifer Nelson, Andy Pearson, Claudia Rogers, Maeve Ryan, Tânia Salgado Pimenta, Carlos Silva Jr., John K. Thornton, and Chaz Yingling.

Many others also contributed in one way or another to this book. Laura Jennings, from the Royal Botanic Gardens, came through when I needed a specialist on West African flora to help me identify the drawing of a medicinal plant made by a British officer while patrolling Atlantic waters.

Emily Berquist, Roquinaldo Ferreira, Toby Green, Katrina Keefer, and William Van Norman Jr. read and commented extensively on the chapters I sent them time and again. Alejandro de la Fuente, Marial Iglesias, and Henry Louis Gates Jr., gave me the opportunity to discuss some of the issues presented in this book on more than one occasion while visiting them in Cambridge, Massachusetts. Likewise, I would struggle to find the appropriate words to thank all the colleagues at the Yale University's Gilder Lehrman Center, from David Blight, who still owes me a Hartford Yard Goats baseball game, to Daniel Vieira, Thomas Thurston and Melissa McGrath, and in particular to my birthday buddy Michelle Zacks and her husband, Eric Applegarth, who made my stay in New Haven really special.

Other friends and colleagues who contributed to this book with conversations, comments, support, etc., are Rosanne Adderley, Vincent Brown, Mariana Candido, Vanja Celevicic, Matt Childs, Adriana Chira, Emma Christopher, Daniel Domingues, Richard Drayton, Marcela Echeverri, Anne Eller, Ada Ferrer, Reinaldo Funes, Louise Gibbs, Alejandro Gómez, Ananya Kabir, Michelle Kelly, David LaFevor, Miranda Lickert, Adrian López, Beatriz Mamigonian, Rafael Marquese, José A. Piqueras, Martín Rodrigo, Matthias Röhrig Assunção, Romy Sánchez, James C. Scott, Randy Sparks, Dale Tomich, Claudia Varella, Christine Whyte, and Michael Zeuske.

Special thanks must go to the personnel of the archives and libraries I visited, sometimes more than once, in Europe, Africa, and the Americas. Without their support and their understanding of the limitations that accompany short, hurried visits, many of the documents I managed to examine would have remained beyond my reach.

My colleagues at the University of Leeds have been forced to listen to my grumbles when doubts came upon me, and to suffer my over-the-top enthusiasm whenever I had a breakthrough or a piece of good news. Particular thanks to Gregorio Alonso, Anyaa Anim-Addo, Nir Arielli, Simon Ball, Alison Fell, Frank Finlay, Bethan Fisk, Sarah Foster, Jan Franklin, Paul Garner, Will Gould, Trudy Green, Simon Hall, Claire Honess, Tom Jackson, Andrea Major, Addi Manolopoulou, Erin Pickles, Alice Potter, Jesús Sanjurjo, Ed Venn, Becky Williams, and Hai-Sui Yu.

At Yale University Press I found a really exceptional crew. From the first meeting I had with Erica Hanson over a coffee at Maison Mathis in New Haven they have been nothing but encouraging and supportive. I have been deeply impressed with their professionalism and expertise. Big thanks are due to Adina Berk, my editor since 2017, whose guidance has been crucial to take this project to the end, I cannot thank her enough for her constant support and encouragement since the first time we exchanged emails. My thanks too to Eva Skewes and particularly Dan Heaton, who have been prompt to answer all of my questions, which have been many, and to offer advice every time I need it.

A final couple of lines to thank my family, and in particular my wife, Effie, and my son, Kenny. Words are not enough to express my gratitude for their being there every day, filling my life with joy and love.

The Yellow Demon of Fever

Introduction

Of what strange nature is knowledge! It clings to the mind,
when it has once seized on it, like a lichen to the rock.

—Mary Wollstonecraft Shelley, *Frankenstein or the
Modern Prometheus* (uncensored 1818 edition)

ON FEBRUARY 22, 1841, Dr. Thomas Nelson boarded a vessel that had
just been escorted into the harbor of Guanabara by HMS *Fawn* under the
command of Lieutenant John Foote. To Nelson, who was already familiar
with the sights, sounds, and scents associated with most slave ships brought
into Rio de Janeiro, this ship, the *Dois de Fevereiro,* seemed remarkably
distinctive. Years later, while recalling the events of that day, he referred to
what he then witnessed as a "loathsome spectacle."[1]

Upon boarding the ship, Nelson observed in horror as more than
360 Africans who had been huddled together on deck—after presumably
being taken from the hold by the crew of the *Fawn*—agonized "with disease, want, and misery stamped upon them with such painful intensity
as utterly beggars all powers of description."[2] Many of them were covered
with the unpleasant abscesses resulting from smallpox infection, and some
were in the last stages of the disease. To compound this dantesque scene,
most of them had "swollen eyelids and the puriform discharge of a virulent
ophthalmia," and were lying around "shrivelled to absolute skin and
bone," all but blind.[3] Evidently affected by this experience, even years later,
Nelson reflected that "deprived of liberty, and torn from their native country, there was nothing more left of human misery but to make them the
victims of a physical darkness as deep as they had already been made of
a moral one."[4]

1

As he walked about deck, the scene turned more and more disturbing, as he discovered a number of mothers with infants who were "vainly endeavouring to suck a few drops of moisture from the[ir] lank, withered, and skinny breasts."[5] Not far from them, he came across the ship sailors, who were also in a sorry state, "suffering from the fever of the coast they had returned from oppressing."[6] One of them in particular, lying almost lifeless, caught his attention, "his lips bloodless, and his countenance wasted and ghastly pale."[7]

After "the first paroxysm of horror and disgust had subsided," Nelson, who was at the time the assistant surgeon on board HMS *Crescent,* a ship moored inside Guanabara harbor in charge of receiving emancipated Africans from slave-trading vessels, began to examine the sick and the dying one by one.[8] Following his own methodology, almost certainly learned in England or Scotland, he started by naming and classifying all the different ailments that affected the Africans and the crew. He concluded that one or more of three diseases—namely smallpox, dysentery, and ophthalmia (probably modern-day trachoma)—were to blame for their afflictions. Other maladies, including skin ulcers, emaciation, and exhaustion, were also responsible for much of the human suffering surrounding him.

Over the following days, Nelson and the personnel of the *Crescent* transferred the vast majority of the Africans to the British ship, now effectively turned into a floating hospital and overcrowded beyond its means with the Africans from the *Dois de Fevereiro,* with others from a second slave ship brought to Rio de Janeiro almost simultaneously, and with the crews of both vessels.[9] With some degree of success, Nelson and his colleagues did everything in their power to treat and revitalize the Africans from the *Dois de Fevereiro.* Although many of them died in the following days as a result of irreversible infections, a month to the date of their capture 180 had recovered sufficiently to reboard the ship and sail under prize officer Gabriel Johnston toward Berbice, where a British Vice-Admiralty court would condemn the ship for participating in the slave trade.[10] Eventually, a few months later, the rest of the surviving Africans would follow their companions as "free laborers" to British Berbice in the steamer *Venezuela.*[11]

Nelson was but one of many men and women who were deeply involved in fighting both the slave trade and its associated diseases in the nineteenth century; a world that came into existence as a direct and immediate result of British foreign policies and practices in the post-1807 Atlantic basin; a world where hurried embarkations and landings, and scant inspection due to time constraints, combined with high-seas battles with navy cruisers, piratical attacks, slave uprisings, and a plethora of previously existing maladies, made the slave trade a much more dangerous and even lethal business. This was especially the case for the African men, women, and children who found themselves bound for the Americas often crammed in the holds of vessels built with the intention of maximizing profits at the expense of human lives and health. In this new world, the respective actions and successes of anti–slave trade patrols and slave traders determined the destinies of all those sold and bought on both sides of the Atlantic, and of those who came into contact with them. More significant, the new dynamics associated with the illegal slave trade contributed to a momentous change in the medical cultures of the Atlantic world; a change that involved new approaches and therapies, as well as new debates about the best ways of controlling diseases, peoples, and geographical spaces.

In this episode, as in many others many times over in this period, Nelson had to diagnose, name, and categorize medical conditions, and to inspect and treat patients, while forecasting the likely course and outcome of their diseases. In other words, like any other health practitioner of the time, he had to use his knowledge to treat his patients to the best of his abilities. From West Africa to Brazil and from the Caribbean to Mozambique, health practitioners—some educated in the universities and colleges of Europe and the Americas and others receptors of conventional knowledge passed down from generation to generation—had to improvise, to keep up with new discoveries and medical developments, to experiment, and to do it all following a trial and error method that frequently caused more harm than the very diseases they were examining and treating. Nelson's personal narrative also illuminates other important issues like the establishment and running of reception centers, hospitals, and lazarettos, and the always-present dilemma of what to do with the bodies of the deceased, particularly those who had died of epidemic diseases.

When the Houses of Parliament in London passed the Abolition of the Slave Trade Act of 1807, the transatlantic slave trade was one of the most

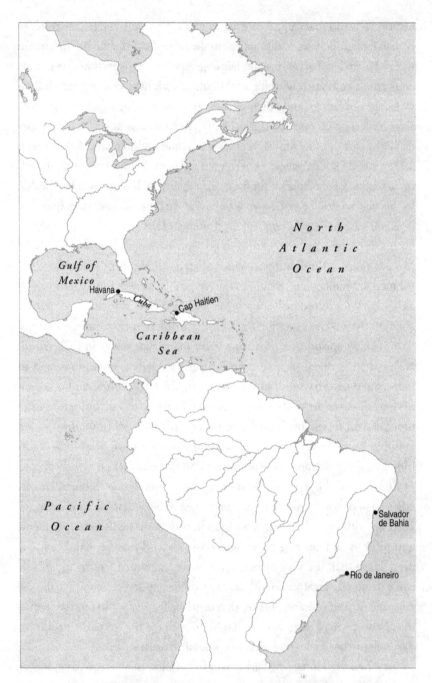

Maps 1 and 2. The Atlantic World in the mid-nineteenth century.

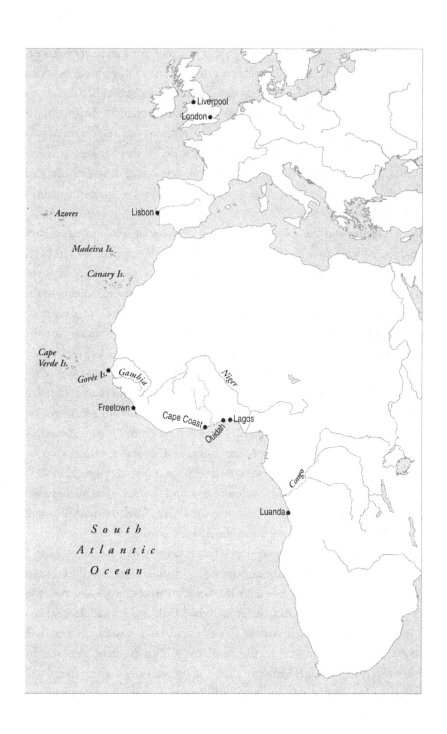

Liverpool
London
Lisbon
Azores
Madeira Is.
Canary Is.
Cape Verde Is.
Gorée Is.
Gambia
Niger
Freetown
Cape Coast
Ouidah
Lagos
Congo
Luanda

South Atlantic Ocean

profitable businesses in the world, but it was one that had never been ex-
empt from difficulties of different sorts throughout its three hundred years
of existence. One of these difficulties was, undoubtedly, that of the dangers
associated with old and new diseases for which the trade in Africa and the
Americas constituted an ideal setting. The removal and relocation of millions of people naturally provoked the creation of new disease environments, and had a profound social, political, economic, demographic, and
epidemiological impact on all those who were involved with this business in
one way or another.[12]

Throughout these centuries, African, European, and American slave
traders, African slaves and their descendants, colonial planters, and at a
later stage anti–slave trade cruiser commanders and crews, were all exposed
to the high morbidity and mortality that accompanied the expansion of the
slave-trading activities from tropical Africa to the Americas. For slave traders and planters it was clear from early on that the loss of human life—the
lives of the slaves—usually equated to a loss of profit, and so, as a norm, they
appear to have endeavored to control, and whenever possible to stop, dangerous diseases from spreading.[13] They did so by taking measures related to
provisioning, diet, and, occasionally, the timing of the Middle Passage. Yet
in truth, medical innovations hardly ever had much to do with the actual
decrease in mortality of slaves, of slave trade and antislaver patrol crews, or
of any other historical actors associated with the traffic. In the hold of slave
vessels, inhumane treatment, overcrowding, and the lack of water and food
were almost certainly the main determinants of the levels of morbidity and
mortality associated with each specific Atlantic crossing.

By the mid-1790s some preventive measures had begun to have a
positive effect on morbidity and mortality rates in the Middle Passage.
This was especially the case after the British Parliament passed the 1788
Slave Trade Regulation Act, better known as Dolben Act, which regulated
the conditions in which African slaves could be acquired, transported,
and treated on their way to the Americas.[14] This positive step and its
effects were irremissibly lost once slave-trading activities became illegal and
began to be conducted in a clandestine manner within the realm of the
illegal Atlantic.[15]

For the enslaved Africans, especially once they had been transplanted to their new destinations in the Americas, staying healthy became of paramount importance for their own survival, so they developed their own medical practices based on their botanical knowledge and understanding of the natural and spiritual worlds that had been passed on to them by their elders, as well as by absorbing new knowledge from their new surroundings.[16] As the Abolition of the Slave Trade Act of 1807 came into effect, British abolitionist efforts in the Atlantic basin led to new approaches and discussions about the diseases associated with the slave trade, which were often based, as Megan Vaughan has suggested, on the conviction that Africa was nothing but "a repository of death, disease, and degeneration, inscribed through a set of recurring and simple dualisms—black and white, good and evil, light and dark."[17] These approaches and discussions, limited as they may have been, did, however, contribute to a major transformation of medical practices from the middle part of the century, and to what Philip D. Curtin has referred to as "a mortality revolution," which also happened to coincide with the dawn of modern epidemiology.[18]

By adopting an intrinsically circum-Atlantic approach, in *The Yellow Demon of Fever* I exhaustively examine the personal experiences of ordinary Atlantic people like Thomas Nelson, who were daily exposed to a wide array of diseases and illnesses, and who were forced to resist and fight them as best as they could, often sharing, intentionally or not, old and new knowledge on the characteristics of these deadly enemies and on how to confront them. I argue that the ways in which these historical actors dealt with and fought against a bewildering array of diseases, how they shared what Pablo Gómez has aptly referred to as a "fragmentary knowledge," and the manner in which their experiences informed the wider public, were central elements in the transformations of medical cultures that took place in the illegal period throughout the Atlantic world.[19]

This book unravels the story of the uninterrupted struggle that took place across the Atlantic, frequently in the shadows, between humans and often terrifying and puzzling diseases; a struggle that generated a vast amount of information at a time when transatlantic means of communication were significantly enhanced.[20] By focusing on this struggle, I seek to demonstrate that while the enforcement of abolitionist policies in the Atlantic contributed to the eventual end of the transatlantic slave trade, it also led to an increase in the suffering of those who were enslaved and sent into the transatlantic slave trade. Thanks to the undoing of policy-related humanitarian advances achieved in the final years of the legal period, which had regulated the conditions aboard British slave ships and the overall manner in which this human traffic was conducted, the patrolling of the Atlantic in this new age stimulated uncontrolled practices carried out in the shadows of illegality, which significantly augmented the ravages of devastating diseases, and human suffering in general.[21]

I also argue that in spite of this step backward, slave traders' worries about the health of their cargoes, as well as anti–slave trade patrol officers' concerns about the health of their prizes—both related to the maximization of profits—generated transatlantic discussions and dialogues about the diseases they encountered and the best ways to fight them, which in turn contributed to the dissemination of old and new knowledge about these diseases, and to palliate, to a certain extent, the detrimental effects on human health of hurried shipping and landing operations, and of overcrowded barracoons—temporary slave prisons—and vessels.

Put in other words, fighting disease was the one goal that all those interested in abolishing the slave trade or involved in keeping it alive as a viable economic activity had in common. As slave traders and those who sought to end their traffic in human beings fought each other, they all found themselves engaged in a common struggle against deadly diseases that did not discriminate among their ranks when selecting their victims. Perhaps as a mixed blessing for those who were enslaved, slave traders and anti–slave trade personnel often did so while trying to keep them alive so that they could sell them in Brazilian and Cuban slave marts, or claim the prize money associated with their release from the hands of the slave traders.

The transatlantic slave trade was a major and expanding activity from the sixteenth century to its final abolition in the second half of the nineteenth century. The trade was a result of initial negotiations between European traders and African rulers, and it grew into a widespread venture involving peoples from three continents, with the Europeans at the helm. Portuguese, Dutch, English, French, and eventually American, Spanish, Cuban, and Brazilian traders settled in West, West Central, and East Africa, opening new markets for the procurement of slaves that were then taken to the Americas to work as field laborers or domestic servants. To a large extent, the transatlantic slave trade was a direct consequence of the Columbian Exchange on the American side of the Atlantic. When the autochthonous Amerindian populations began to be wiped out by brutal oppression and European diseases for which they had no immunity, European colonizers were faced with what Alfred Crosby has referred to as "the greatest labor shortage of all time."[22]

As a result, African laborers were sought to replace them, leading to another "exchange" along the coasts of the African continent, one in which the Europeans seem to have come—in epidemiological terms—second best.[23] The transatlantic slave trade was thus nothing short of a mammoth challenge that provoked new ideas, but also new fears and anxieties that were apparent not only along the "dreaded" African coast but also in Europe and the Americas. At a time when vaccines were in their infancy and antibiotics were nonexistent, the prevalent belief in "the acquired and, in some cases, genetic resistance of native Africans to these diseases" constituted a pivotal element in the growth of the transatlantic trade in human beings.[24] Likewise, fears of contagion, which presented tropical regions as dangerous repositories of disease, were rooted in the European imperial encounter with colonial bodies, which in their opinion had to be policed, enlightened, and cured. This "need" then offered them "scientific" and moral justifications to define racial boundaries that invariably presented whites as masters who offered civilization and the true god, and nonwhites as savages, ignorants, idolaters, and so on.

The indispensable interactions between European, African, and American peoples originated and developed within what Marie Louise Pratt has referred to as contact zones, where tropical disease became an unsuspected and lethal trading item. In these contact zones, smallpox, yellow fever, malaria, typhoid fever, dysentery, and many other afflictions were transmitted and, as a result, were also spread across the Atlantic basin. The white man's grave, as many different parts of West Africa were known, was the grave not only of Europeans but also of many an African, and the slave trade—both on land and at sea—was the most adept activity for the propagation of these diseases among distant places and peoples.

It was in these contact zones where a process of transculturation—involving disease, as well as European, African, and American medical research and practices—took place.[25] According to Pratt, these contact zones were a "space of colonial encounters," where "peoples geographically and historically separated come into contact with each other and established ongoing relations, usually involving conditions of coercion, radical inequality, and intractable conflict."[26] Slave factories and other European settlements, vessels of various kinds—especially those transporting slaves—and American cities and plantations that served as destination for the men, women, and children enslaved and displaced from their homes, were all textbook contact zone examples. As a matter of fact, it would not be far-fetched to talk about slave-trade contact zones—a term I use extensively in the pages of this book—as a specific type of contact zones, centered around human trafficking, and with its own parameters and characteristics.

Indeed, both Pratt and Crosby, as well as many other contemporary scholars, have emphasized the human cost of these exchanges. Crosby, who in his foundational 1972 book *The Columbian Exchange: Biological and Cultural Consequences of 1492* focused predominantly on the American side of these interactions, placed both ecological disaster and death at the core of his study.[27] When discussing the ways in which Amerindian peoples were affected by the arrival of Old World humans, he went as far as stating that irrespective of whether Europeans and Africans "came to the native Americans in war or peace, they always brought death with them."[28] Disease and death were ever-present hostile entities, often described by practitioners, authors, and people in general with anthropomorphic epithets and humanlike personalities.[29] They inhabited these contact zones alongside humans, and, even on those occasions when they were not present, they were still feared and considered likely to strike at any point.

Understanding how these diseases were transmitted and how their ravages could be contained became issues of crucial importance for the success of slave-trading enterprises, abolitionist efforts, and ultimately of colonialism itself. There were several lines of argument in defining what provoked these diseases and what were the best and most effective ways of combating them. In simple terms, it could be argued that there was an ontological clash of sorts among miasma theory enthusiasts, who argued that diseases were likely to be the product of poisonous vapors resulting from decomposing matter; humoralists, who pinned their understanding of disease on the ancient theory of the four body fluids; followers of the homeopathic method proposed by German practitioner Samuel Hahnemann, in which the "law of the similars" came to have a central stage; community morals controllers, like preachers and missionaries, who saw human behavior as central to any issue related to how diseases were acquired and treated; and, finally, those very few who at the time were beginning to contend that many of these diseases were in fact transmitted from person to person by vector carriers of microorganisms. Their points of view were not always exclusive, as the debates between contagionists and anticontagionists sustained for most of the first half of the nineteenth century demonstrated. The various ways of understanding disease exhibited by every Atlantic actor during this period were fundamental for determining the measures that could be taken in order to control disease-ridden environments—just like people, environments were often considered to be sick, and subsequently became the subjects of prophylactic measures, treatments, and cures—and to stop epidemics and other diseases from spreading.

Nevertheless, these measures had consistently little impact, at least from an epidemiological point of view. The various characteristics of the diseases practitioners had to deal with, and the intrinsically speculative element in their approaches often resulted in very limited degrees of success and in high levels of human suffering. The variety and the number of diseases were overwhelming for all those who came in contact with them. There were endemic ones and epidemic ones; curable ones and incurable ones; some that were highly contagious and infectious, and others that were not.[30] Such uncertainty led British surgeon Robert Clarke to comment that this variety of diseases constituted "a great difficulty" for health practitioners in West Africa, as they attempted to "apply remedies" in spite of the almost total "impossibility of their arriving at a true diagnosis."[31] Additionally, it should not be forgotten that the diverse disorders of the mind, often associated with the traumatic experience of the Middle Passage, were habitually found alongside all other diseases. In some cases, as happened in the first half of the nineteenth century in Sierra Leone, they were so devastating that local authorities had no option but to create wards or hospitals specifically intended for psychiatric patients.[32]

Meanwhile, as Alan Bewell has stated, back in Europe, in the supposedly civilized world, "major cultural myths" were built on the differences between these diseases and their effects on people of different sexes, races, and cultural backgrounds. Differences in the anatomy and physiology of men and women, as well as those of adults, the elderly, and children, signaled the efforts to understand and curtail disease in the Atlantic slave trade.[33] Even more relevant were the differences in the reactions to particular infections and specific treatments shown by white and black men and women. As we have seen, the alleged tolerance of Africans to the severity of tropical climates—and its associated diseases—was from very early on an important excuse for their enslavement in Africa and their transplantation to the Americas.[34]

Although this was not by any means always the case, the ways of fighting these diseases were frequently determined by fragmentary mismatched pieces of knowledge anchored in myths, as well as by the lack of understanding of what they were dealing with, which often rendered them perplexed. A case in question, albeit from an earlier period, is that of seventeenth-century Havana, whose residents were repeatedly visited by epidemics of yellow fever, measles, typhus, and smallpox. The city's Cabildo, or council, powerless to fight these epidemics, often reverted to intensive praying as the only way to stop them from causing further ravages. In 1637, faced with simultaneous deathly outbreaks of smallpox and measles that were killing "the old and the young, [and] the white and the black," they convened in early February and proposed to have a public praying session to the Lord and a procession in honor of Saint Sebastian and Saint Roque, to invoke their intercession.[35] Similar proposals were made in September 1667, when typhus attacked the city again, and in 1676 after another outbreak of smallpox decimated its population one more time.[36] What the Cabildo and citizens of Havana experienced at the time was in all ways representative of the fears, anxieties, and limited medical knowledge existing at the time everywhere across the Atlantic. Two centuries later, as governments on both sides of the Atlantic endeavored to put in place public health measures which included bills of health, quarantines, inoculation, and vaccination to counteract the ravages of disease, superstitious practices and religious prayers continued to coexist with these measures in what Vincent Brown has referred to as "an enchanted world."[37]

In addition to prayers and processions, Europeans, Africans, and Americans were forced to experiment with different theories and practices, relying on a trial-and-error method for most of the period, until some scientific breakthroughs were finally made in the second half of the nineteenth century. Of the major killers, only three were somehow brought under control from the final years of the eighteenth century thanks to contemporary innovations, although it is worth pointing out that they continued to affect those involved in the slave trade until its very end in the latter part of the 1860s. Smallpox, after the inoculation method and the variolic vaccine were made available to slave traders and health practitioners throughout the Atlantic, was fought with at least some degree of success. This was particularly the case among Westerners who had had easier access to the vaccine for years.[38] Scurvy was largely resolved when it became apparent that fruits with a high concentration of vitamin C, like oranges and lemons, were effective in diminishing and even eradicating the malady, while malarial fevers were, for the first time, being fought across the Atlantic with an improved degree of success thanks to the ever-increasing and more appropriate use of Peruvian bark or sulfate of quinine.[39]

Determining how to fight fevers and other maladies was equally a difficult task, especially considering the varied nomenclature that some of them had at the time. Just to cite one among several examples: fevers as a category comprised, among many others, yellow fever (also known as black vomit, bulam fever, and *typhus icterodes*), malaria (remittent fever, recurrent fever, intermittent fever), dengue fever (break bone fever), typhus (ship fever, hospital fever), and typhoid fever (slow fever, nervous fever, intermittent fever).

The documents produced by those who came into contact with them reflect plenty of doubts, and wide-ranging and vague classifications often led to unreliable projections with regard to the course that they could take in each specific patient. Although in some cases a fatal outcome was almost certain, as with African human trypanosomiasis (sleeping sickness), in others survival and even full recovery were to be expected.

All the practitioners' efforts, forlorn as they may have seemed, were not without hope; at least this was the case in what related to the provision of care and therapy. Medical doctors, surgeons, and healers across the Atlantic did their best in trying different solutions and remedies to improve the health of those under their care, often following the advice of medical manuals and journals, which are discussed in the pages of this book, or following the recommendations of local practitioners who had had certain degrees of success in fighting these maladies.

Eventually the diagnosis, prognosis, and treatment of each of these afflictions took central stage in the historical record resulting from four centuries of human trafficking in the Atlantic world. The contributions made by Africans, European traders and surgeons, New World planters and medical doctors, and many others, produced a medical corpus that led to the constant interrogation of the causes of these diseases and to a better understanding of a number of aspects associated with them.

In this battle, the role of public policy was often decisive, as the protection of population groups was deemed to be of the highest importance.[40] In this manner, for example, the old recourse to quarantines became instrumental for the provision of isolation establishments in the face of looming epidemics.[41] Throughout the Atlantic, other old measures that had been repeatedly used over the centuries to fight disease were reproduced. Reception centers, lazarettos, and hospitals, often located outside urban limits, provided the necessary setting for the separation of the sick and the healthy in the aftermath of British abolition. On various occasions, hospital vessels were preferred, as they could be kept even farther away from local, healthy populations. Funeral practices too were altered accordingly, following practices that had begun to be employed in previous centuries. For instance, in several of the Atlantic locations featured in this book, cemeteries were relocated to rural areas in order to bury those who had died of contagious or infectious diseases away from heavily populated centers.

The Africans received by Thomas Nelson on that fateful day of February 1841, as well as the crew of the ship that took them across the ocean, were all part of an illegal Atlantic culture that had proliferated in the aftermath of the Abolition of the Slave Trade Act of 1807, and in particular after the first bilateral abolitionist treaties began to come into effect in 1820. This illegal Atlantic culture was nothing but a logical sequel of prior historical periods in which smuggling, piracy, and contraband had created similar concealed environments where covert transactions were the norm, and where illicitness was a means to an end.[42] Intrinsically related to the illegal continuation of the slave trade after 1807, this badly studied milieu was populated by a wide array of ordinary actors who included those who were enslaved, as well as those who coordinated, carried out, serviced, and fought human traffic in the Atlantic world and beyond.

In their seminal book *The Many-Headed Hydra: The Hidden History of the Revolutionary Atlantic,* first published in 2000, Peter Linebaugh and Marcus Rediker had already hinted, even in the title, at the existence of an early modern Atlantic world where a revolutionary, proletarian, anticapitalist culture had emerged at the margins of rising merchant capitalism.[43] The men and women Linebaugh and Rediker referred to as "outcasts of all nations," quoting an English colonial officer in the Caribbean, continued to exist in the Atlantic world during the age of abolition, although during this period they frequently carried out their undertakings in tandem with slave dealers and corrupt authorities.[44] Their existence, however, was much challenged and changed by new circumstances, which were mostly determined by the commitment of the British authorities to pursue and punish the transatlantic slave trade, particularly after 1820.

Certainly, many of them continued to carry out similar activities in the shadows, often living their lives in anonymity and in relative isolation. Others, however, thanks to the protection given to them by local African rulers and Spanish, Portuguese, and Brazilian authorities, lived lives that were not as concealed—some of them even attaining titles of nobility—and left a trail of written historical evidence thanks to which we can now, to a certain extent, reconstruct their existence.[45]

Given the involvement of the British government and navy in the abolition of the slave trade in the post-1807 period, it is not surprising that a considerable number of primary sources on the illegal Atlantic were produced precisely by those British Royal Navy and consular officers, settlers, and missionaries. British abolitionist actors in the Atlantic, including Mixed Commission and Vice-Admiralty courts personnel, Royal Navy commanders and sailors, and a number of missionaries, travelers, and explorers of diverse origins, left remarkable written accounts of their activities and journeys. Their constant interactions with slaves, slave dealers, and other associated actors—think of Nelson's description of the slaves and crew members of the *Dois de Fevereiro*—also turned them into important actors and witnesses of this Atlantic underworld. Other important primary accounts of the events and issues discussed in this book were produced by Spanish, French, Portuguese, Brazilian, and American authorities, anti–slave trade personnel, merchants, and a diverse range of peoples who came into contact with the slave-trade contact zones during this period.

Each of these groups of actors counted among its ranks health practitioners, who were daily exposed to bewildering diseases and the human suffering that, more often than not, accompanied them. The term *health practitioners* is used throughout this book while referring to this assortment of medical men and women, in order to avoid unnecessary nomenclatures that would serve only to stress the differences between Europeans, Africans, and Americans. Alternative terminologies are used only in some specific cases, where practitioners are referred to by their titles (for example, colonial surgeon, *sangrador,* or Mallam).

The struggles of these practitioners, and those who collaborated with them in their efforts to care and treat their patients and to understand these diseases, were not, however, evenly chronicled for posterity. As often happens, the work of American and European practitioners and their collaborators—even in the less obvious cases of lawless slave traders—were better documented than that of their African counterparts. What little we know about African medical and botanical knowledge during this period has reached us precisely thanks to European and American physicians, colonial officers, explorers, missionaries, and travelers, who took care to note down, with different degrees of interest, detail, and accuracy, what they had observed and learned during their interactions with African men, women, and children.[46] Bringing these African and African-descended practitioners into the fold of this research has been an uphill battle from the start, as the overwhelming majority of the sources featuring their work and knowledge were produced by Westerners who were more often than not full of praise for their own methods, practices, and knowledge while belittling the contributions of the African practitioners they met.

Problematic as they may be, these historical sources can nonetheless help us elucidate the ways in which diseases were fought within the realm of the post-1807 illicit slave trade. At times, they also offer a window into how public health efforts served as a back door for the ever-increasing expansion of colonial and imperial interests and for the stereotyping, often negative, of non-Western peoples and cultures. Notably, they also reveal human doubts, fears, and anxieties; experimental treatments; and empirical recollection, regurgitation, framing, and transfer of new and old ways of fighting disease.

It is worth mentioning one final aspect related to the pitfalls of studies focusing on the medical history of the slave trade. Until now, most of the existing research about medical knowledge, and the struggle against disease in the slave trade, has broadly concentrated on the licit and better-documented pre-1807 period. The many works produced for this period have addressed not only diseases and their cures but also mortality and morbidity rates, and on occasion have centered on the medical profession, looking squarely at the work of Atlantic surgeons.[47]

Studies of the interactions between humans and the diseases confronted in the post-1807 transatlantic slave trade are less forthcoming, in spite of this world having served as a propitious background to many of the medical debates of the period, and being the setting where many drugs and therapies were developed and tested time and again. To date only a limited number of authors have attempted to shed light on issues such as morbidity and mortality rates, provision of medical services aboard slave ships, and related topics for which studies on the previous centuries are abundant.[48] This lack of truly transatlantic studies on the medical history of the post-1807 illegal slave trade is probably a result of its very concealed nature, and of the methodological and practical challenges presented to anyone interested in studying the topic, which include, but are not limited to, doing research in a considerable number of archives, libraries, and repositories from the three continents involved in this history, and often having to read and interpret documents written in several different languages. That the primary sources used in this book are spread across several countries should not surprise anyone, as the actors involved in the story told in its pages were nothing short of a truly international, circum-Atlantic cast. One of the main challenges undertaken in the following pages has been to cast these sources "in a new geographical framework," while drawing from the histories of the transatlantic slave trade and medicine, as well as colonialism and imperialism.[49] Ultimately, such a methodological approach allows for an emphasis on the stories of the ordinary peoples who are at the core of this study, who met one another, and who confronted one another's fears, anxieties, and diseases throughout the Atlantic world.

Furthermore, almost all studies produced on the topic of medicine and slavery for this period to date have had a self-imposed cis-Atlantic focus—to use David Armitage's terminology—and most have been based on cases drawn from the U.S. antebellum South or from the British American territories, often focusing on slavery in rural and urban settings rather than on the actual transatlantic slave traffic.[50] Only recently, some innovative studies have begun to appear, mostly in Brazil, examining a number of aspects of the veiled universe of medical practitioners, chiefly Africans, in the illegal Atlantic world.[51]

I purposely refrain in *The Yellow Demon of Fever* from focusing exclusively on the romantic image of the Western "civilized" practitioner fighting disease against all the odds within alien environments that often were nothing short of "disaster zones."[52] Instead, I seek to reveal the extent to which African and African-descended practitioners also contributed to this struggle. Overall, health practitioners and other witnesses of this epic battle against deathly and debilitating diseases, upon whose knowledge and documented practices this book rests, came from different walks of life. Many of them were characters living at the margins of the law, including many African practitioners as well as shady slave-ship and factory surgeons. Others carried out their works in an open and legal manner, even though on occasion they were also involved in the slave trade or in its suppression.

Western travelers, colonists, missionaries, slave dealers, and anti-slave trade patrol personnel bequeathed to us most of the existing historical material, including that pertaining to Africans' knowledge and practices. The vast majority are short accounts of encounters with Africans, in which they—both men and women—were often described with pejorative terms like juju men, witch doctors, fake healers, charlatans, and the like. With some glaring exceptions, these accounts all focus on African local medical practices based on the practitioners' knowledge of local botany and customary treatments. By no means a new phenomenon, some of this African medical knowledge continued to be taken across the Atlantic to resurface again, fragmented and modified, in the cities and on the plantations of the Americas where European or American observers often referred to it with awe, surprised by its effectiveness.[53]

Slave-ship, slave-port, and factory practitioners dwelled in an even more ambiguous realm. They carried out their work on slave vessels crammed with sick enslaved Africans, regularly plagued by epidemic diseases, or had no remedy but to settle down in West, West Central, or East African coastal villages and towns where tropical diseases were endemic, frequently losing their health or lives in their attempts to make small fortunes. Until now we have learned very little about this assortment of physicians, surgeons, and other practitioners, but thanks to a number of sources never or rarely used before, they, too, are central characters in the story that this book tells.

In spite of their often-direct links with the slave trade, significant numbers of ordinary health practitioners in places like the French Caribbean, Cuba, Puerto Rico, the antebellum South, and Brazil were, more often than not, recognized by their fellow practitioners. Their relationship with recently arrived Africans yielded a number of written texts of various quality and length. These treaties, accounts, and memoirs, which were a result of the authors' own experiments in tackling the diseases discussed here, also occasionally included accounts of remedies and practices they had learned from the same men and women they were charged with taking care of. The literature produced by these practitioners, particularly in the West Indies, but also in Brazil and other Atlantic localities, circulated widely among colleagues in Europe and the Americas. In some cases, these books and shorter pamphlets served to determine not just how to deal with sick slaves but also how to provide healthier environments that could eventually lead to bigger margins of profits, as well as the expansion and consolidation of new colonial outposts.[54]

Anti–slave trade patrols and colonial practitioners, as well as medical officers who settled or traveled across the Atlantic during this period for different reasons, also had the opportunity to write down their experiences and observations. In a number of cases, they went as far as publishing them, at once furthering their own professional careers and providing newly arrived physicians with valuable accounts of their experiences and knowledge. Some of these treaties became nothing short of precious practical manuals offering all sorts of advice on how to combat the diseases associated to the illicit slave trade, and were frequently cited as the foremost authorities in the field.

Far away from the European and American centers of power, the illicit slave trade presented medical practitioners and their collaborators with opportunities to test and trial old and new therapies. The lack of rigorous control led to practices that were often plainly disastrous. During a period known today as the Age of Heroic Medicine across the Western world, medical practitioners in the illegal Atlantic world took these experiments, including the use of mercury, bloodletting, and purgatives, to an entire new level of reckless vigor in search of chimeric results.[55]

Although such strategies always represented a last resort to save lives when faced with unpredictable life-threatening diseases, enslaved Africans were used routinely, with little difficulty, in the trial and testing of scientific and not-so-scientific treatments. From the time they were captured and taken to the African coast to wait for embarkation, they were subjected not only to deadly or weakening maladies but also to medical treatments that frequently had more damaging results than the symptoms they were supposed to remedy. Their situation, if anything, deteriorated during the Middle Passage, where being crammed into small, dark, hot, humid, and dirty spaces, in which epidemics ravaged entire human groups, led to more of the same deathly dichotomy of disease and treatment.

But enslaved Africans were not the only ones who suffered at the hands of the medical practitioners. Captains and crews of slave vessels, slave dealers settled along the African coast, anti–slave trade patrol crews, and the local inhabitants of each of these Atlantic ports and slave factories were equally subjected to drugs and treatments that were often lethal. Their stories of despair and suffering, like those of the Africans they came into contact with, are also told in the pages of this book.

In the words of Laura T. Murphy, "The practice of sacrificing human lives for the sake of material gain is a legacy of the devastating devaluation of human life that was integral to the workings of the slave trade."[56] Although Murphy's powerful words would resonate with anyone studying virtually any aspect of the transatlantic slave trade and its short-, medium-, and long-term consequences, they are particularly appropriate to refer to the sort of human trafficking that developed after the British began enforcing their abolitionist policies across the Atlantic, forcing slave traders to go to unprecedented lengths to conceal their activities. In this new age, the value of human lives, especially those of the Africans, was trivial. The business of the slave trade had to carry on regardless, and so it did. Within this vicious new realm of illicit trade in human beings, splattered with disease and death, medical knowledge turned into an essential tool in the hands of nearly every person with the capabilities to treat the infirm and the sick.

After being forced by anti–slave trade patrols to rush their human cargoes without all the health checks that had been more frequent in the legal, pre-1807 period, slave traders wisely did everything in their power to learn and disseminate the most advanced ways of dealing with the diseases of the slave trade. African slaves, those who enslaved them in the Americas, and the various British and other European and American practitioners, officers, sailors, and travelers who came into contact with them did the same.

After all, these fatal diseases were their common, and certainly their most dangerous, enemies. Medical knowledge, then, became a weapon of sorts, not just because it served to fight back against diseases that were considered to be lethal foes, but also because it facilitated the maximization of profits obtained from every human cargo.

Medical knowledge, however, was not always homogeneous or effective. The descriptions we have inherited from those who lived in, or at the margins of, the illegal Atlantic, are probably just as varied. In spite of the fact that they all had vested interests in what can only be described as early colonial endeavors, specialized practitioners were able to document experiments, therapies, and epidemics—to mention but a few examples of recordable actions and events—in scientific ways that missionaries or travelers were not, as their interests often drifted toward moral, religious, and other nonmedical matters. In this respect, their writings provided precious intelligence in the renewed attempts at trading with and colonizing Africa. At opposite ends of this spectrum and illustrating this point are the reports of two notable residents of Freetown in the early nineteenth century: colonial surgeon James Boyle and Methodist missionary Reverend William Davies, 1st.[57]

In 1831, upon his return to England from West Africa, where he had served for years as the colonial surgeon of Sierra Leone, James Boyle published his magnum opus, a medical treaty entitled *A Practical Medico-Historical Account of the Western Coast of Africa*. The book was one of the first to provide some sort of utilitarian text that could serve the practical purposes of health practitioners, residents, and travelers along the coast of Africa, and in the wider Atlantic world. The first few lines of the book's introduction were a robust reminder to his colleagues about the lack of medical treatises—and reliable knowledge—specifically destined to address the tropical diseases that affected the inhabitants of West Africa and those who visited the region in almost equal measure. "It is not little extraordinary in these days of unparalleled thirst for knowledge," he lamented, "that no work, until the present, has been attempted, specifically upon the Diseases of Western Africa."[58]

On the other extreme of the spectrum, Reverend William Davies 1st, who was the first Welsh Methodist minister to travel to Sierra Leone to spread the gospel, published an account in which his missionary activity was mixed with the firsthand experiences during his time in the West African British colony. Davies, like every other visitor to West or West Central Africa during the period, felt compelled to recount the deadly atmosphere and landscape surrounding him, but because of his own role, a considerable part of his narrative, as well as some of his letters written just before he sailed for West Africa, are focused on the missionary work he had undertaken, and on the moral hazards he saw everywhere he went.[59]

For men like Boyle and Davies, Africa was a new frontier that needed to be politically, religiously, and medically conquered and colonized. They were the standard bearers of a new wave of European and American men and women who considered their incipient colonialist and capitalist ideas as righteous on their own, and central to the future of Africa and the wider world.[60] Although collaboration was often the norm, they were also frequently opposed by a collection of random people that included Africans, slave traders, and all those with an interest in the continuation of the trade, including the governments of Portugal, Spain, and Brazil, among others. Among this latter group, colonialist and emerging capitalist ideas were just as common as they were among men like Boyle and Davies. In their attempts to justify their illegal engagement in human trafficking ventures, they often resorted to arguing the need for "civilizing" and Christianizing Africa and the Africans, habitually portraying themselves as the natural and needed saviors of the very people they were enslaving and uprooting from their homes, and whose lands they were buying cheap or taking by force.[61]

Just as religious men like Davies were needed to pacify and convert "uncivilized" Africans, health practitioners like Boyle were essential for the necessary operations of new European settlements. Without them, mercantile capitalist enterprises and the nascent colonialism of the early nineteenth century that was determined to open Africa to Western businesses would not have been possible. This proposition also applied to those practitioners who settled and made possible the functioning of illicit slave-trading ports and factories along the African coast, and who traveled back and forth across the Atlantic taking care of the human cargoes of those who had hired them.

Virtually every European or American settlement along the African coast, regardless of its relationship with the slave trade, counted at least one health practitioner—African, European, or American—in charge of fighting disease. The same applied to all vessels, independent of whether they were engaged in human traffic or in its repression. Health practitioners, even those who were enslaved Africans, were leading lights of the post-1807 illegal Atlantic cast, regardless of their respective places of birth, gender, skin color, social status, or religious, political, and economic allegiances.

Sometime after finishing his consular appointment at the British diplomatic mission in Rio de Janeiro, where he had worked alongside doctors Nelson and Gunn for a few years in the 1830s and 1840s, William Gore Ouseley felt compelled, as Nelson had before, to publish a volume discussing the slave trade to Brazil. The book, published in 1850 and entitled *Notes on the Slave-Trade with Remarks on the Measures Adopted for its Suppression,* dealt with a wide array of issues pertaining to the illegal traffic of human beings from Africa to Brazil, and was based mostly on his firsthand experiences dealing with slave traders and Brazilian authorities.

Although Ouseley was not a health practitioner, he included a few remarks on the diseases brought to Brazil from the coast of Africa, reaching some significant conclusions about their impact on the chances of success of slave-trading expeditions, and for the eventual end of the slave trade in the Atlantic world. To be sure, and echoing French physician Matthieu Audouard's theories, Ouseley established a direct link between the transatlantic slave trade and the transmission of infectious malaises when he pointed out that disease "frequently becomes either a check on the Slave-trade or its punishment, for at this moment the yellow fever, or some equally fatal epidemic, that rages at Rio de Janeiro and elsewhere in Brazil, serves to show at what a risk the Slave-trade is carried on."[62]

At the time Ouseley wrote these words in the late 1840s, health practitioners and ordinary people echoed them publicly and privately throughout the Atlantic world. By then, every single person involved in this illegal business was well aware of the dangers associated with trafficking human beings against their wishes across the ocean. Alongside the always threatening sight of anti–slave trade patrol cruisers and the latent likelihood of having to face an African uprising while at sea, potentially devastating diseases needed to be factored in every time a slave vessel departed for a transatlantic voyage. The situation was similar in factories and ports on both sides of the Atlantic, where diseases often determined public policy, international relations, and colonialist agendas.

In another part of his narrative, Ouseley reflected, not without reason, that while "in pursuit of his victims the slave-trader does not hesitate to sacrifice human life in the most reckless manner."[63] In this unruly and brutal world, human life had little or no value, a circumstance that was not, however, irreconcilable with the fact that trading in enslaved Africans was at its most profitable when the human cargoes were delivered on the American side of the ocean in good health. It is not surprising that efforts were made throughout the period to carry as many healthy men, women, and children across the Atlantic as possible. Fighting disease was, then, a crucial occupation among slave traders, just as it was among those attempting to suppress their activities, as in many cases recaptured Africans represented a sum of money for those who had seized and taken them before any of the Atlantic courts of the period.

Natural environments, like people, often needed to be treated and cured, as for many they constituted the principal source of the maladies that affected settlements along the African coast, slave vessels, and the urban and rural areas where African slaves were taken and forced to work as slaves. To this end, renewed efforts were made by the collection of Atlantic actors studied in the pages of this book, to identify, name, and treat these diseases, often following pieces of healing knowledge inherited from European, African, and American sources whose origins were diverse and which had various degrees of success.

The latter years of the transatlantic slave trade provided a perfect stage for this ongoing battle between humans and pathogens. This was a battleground where diseases were still overpowering, and where an imprecise and fragmented medical knowledge was the best weapon available in the hands of practitioners and other Atlantic actors, who did their best to rein in the devastating effects of these maladies. They did so in what was, by any measure, an environment shrouded by apprehension, where ordinary people lived in constant fear of contracting one of the many diseases that inhabited these contact zones; an environment where, as Robert Jameson, the first British Mixed Commission judge in Havana, reflected, "the yellow demon of fever" always glared "terrifically at them."[64]

ONE

"A Beautiful Spot for a Grave"

Prophylaxis and Prevention in the
Slave-Trade Contact Zones

I'll rove where the tropical forests lie darkling
For bright things there buried like flowers with the dead;
I'll search where the sands of bright rivers are sparkling,
That o'er thee those wonders and gems may be shed.
—David Francis Bacon, *Wanderings on the Seas and Shores of Africa*

UPON HIS ARRIVAL in Freetown to act as a Spanish official in the newly created Anglo-Spanish Mixed Commission Court of Sierra Leone in 1819, Spanish judge José Camps was attacked by the famous fever of the country, considered fatal for most of those Europeans who dared to venture along the West African coastline. In a despairing letter sent to Spain's secretary of state, Carlos Martínez de Yrujo, Marquis of Casa Yrujo, Camps described his predicament, pointing out that he found himself writing "from a hospital, or more appropriately, from a cemetery."[1] Camps then recounted in detail that the burning fevers had grown larger as the "rains, incessant since the beginnings of June till the end of October" had set in. In Camps's own words, of the 118 Europeans that had been living in Freetown at the time of his arrival, 53 had already died.[2]

Camps's fears of dying in such a short time were neither new nor unfounded, as all European settlements along the coast had been devastated repeatedly by a combination of diseases, against which their medicinal remedies and medical therapies usually proved hopeless. In fact, all across the

27

Atlantic world, slaves, soldiers, sailors, anti–slave trade patrols' personnel, merchants, health practitioners, and a host of related characters struggled against devastating diseases they could not often control or cure. The continuous effort in identifying, naming, and classifying these maladies was in itself a gargantuan challenge.

In this chapter I grapple with a number of issues associated with how these diseases were perceived across the Atlantic world and what ideas and methods were recommended and devised to prevent their arrival and dissemination. One central preventative objective was how to sanitize ships, buildings, and other trading areas, in order to reduce the threat that so-called pestilential environments posed to all those who came into contact with them; another was the need to regulate human behavior so as to prevent the spread of disease. Both objectives were coincidentally convenient for the proliferation of Western settlements along the African shores. The goal of stopping the spread of diseases allowed for the implementation of a number of measures, which also had the effect of preventing African populations from challenging the power of European and American officers on land and at sea. The decisions and policies of European and American actors on the African coast, however, were also influenced by discussions that took place all over the Atlantic world and beyond during the period.

These discussions regularly included health practitioners, politicians, and a variety of other actors, each of them with his or her own agenda. Predictably, in an age where Western powers ruled the Atlantic, the results of these debates had a direct impact on the development of capitalist ventures and protocolonial projects. Because of the permanent presence of lethal and debilitating diseases, Western medical knowledge constituted an ever-present trait in this process. However, the limitations of that medical knowledge implicitly challenged the supposed superiority of Western actors whenever they came into contact with their African counterparts, especially in Africa. This presence was particularly observable as proponents and opponents of continuing and expanding the slave trade carved their respective niches along the African coast through negotiation, deception, and force. In the contact zones of the illegal slave trade in the 1800s, human traffickers and their British, French, American, and Portuguese nemeses all had to confront deadly and enervating environments and diseases, and all took advantage of diplomatic and military interventions to exert their claims over lands and peoples, not only in Africa but also in the Americas and even at sea.

How did local authorities, slave dealers, health practitioners, missionaries, anti–slave trade squadron captains, and others attempt to prevent and control the diseases to which they were exposed in the slave-trade contact zones? By looking at how they understood the prevailing miasma theory and the need to regulate human humors and behaviors, and at how their old and new knowledge circulated, we can reach a more in-depth understanding of how diseases were culturally interpreted. Such an analysis can reveal that slave traders and those representing the abolitionist efforts across the Atlantic, under the veil of alleged hygienic containment, used regulations in order to hide their own embryonic expansionist colonial ambitions.

Tropical Diseases in the Slave-Trade Contact Zones

As abolitionist policies were implemented throughout the Atlantic, while Western health practitioners, navy personnel, government officers, and merchants, travelers, and settlers increased their interactions with Africa and its peoples, the already dread-inducing image of the continent they carried with them became more and more apparent. Narratives like those left by Horatio Bridge in the late 1840s infiltrated the imagination of Europeans and Americans, presenting an African continent that was mysterious, rich, exotic, and fatal. When describing Sierra Leone, Bridge could not help resorting to what was perhaps the most popular moniker to denote the African regions where Europeans were all too often the victims of fevers, dysentery, smallpox, and a number of other diseases. Mixing the infamous "White Man's Grave" sobriquet with a fascination—shared by many others—for the lush and picturesque green hills that surrounded Freetown, Bridge referred to what he saw with his eyes as "a beautiful spot for a grave," one that was "as lovely as [an] ornamental cemeter[y]."[3]

Of course, Bridge, like many others, was aware that coming into close proximity to those same charming green hills carried a well-documented

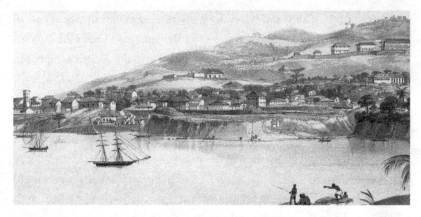

Fig. 1. Freetown c. 1850, with Queen's Yard for Liberated Africans at the center. Auguste François Laby and Jonathan Needham. Courtesy of the Yale Center for British Art, Yale University.

risk of contracting one or more of those dreaded diseases. Since Europeans had settled in places like Sierra Leone, Bissau, Cacheu, and the Gold Coast, and along the Angolan coast, the fear of succumbing to these diseases had been amply presented and discussed among European and American publics in a variety of ways that included government reports, private and official correspondence, and travelers' accounts. These discussions were often accompanied by elaborate descriptions of the adverse circumstances they had to endure, including a lack of basic hygiene and the prevalent filth that existed in the places where they had settled.

In a dispatch dated September 20, 1828, Sierra Leone Acting Governor Samuel Smart referred to the unfavorable conditions of the streets of Freetown during the rainy season, observing that the continuous rains left them exposed to dangerous floods that carried loose earth, forming "deep and very dangerous gutters and channels in every street."[4] This situation led Governor Smart to argue before the Town Council that macadamization of the streets should be undertaken immediately to arrest the spreading of disease during this season. Up the coast, in the Gambia, hazards were similar. Two years before Governor Smart's missive, Assistant Surgeon John Bell reported that during the rainy season most of Bathurst's streets had to be "cut in the centre to permit the water to flow from the houses, bearing a resemblance to many rivulets running their courses."[5] Another colleague, William Ferguson, while discussing the situation around the British settlements on the Gold Coast, too mentioned what he considered "the filthiness of the villages" in the vicinity of their forts in Accra and Cape Coast.[6] Similarly, upon returning to the United States from Africa in 1836, Charles Hoffman pointed out to the secretary of the navy that "the filthiness of the inhabitants and the vicinity of low marshes" had contributed to the injurious character of the Portuguese settlement in Bissau.[7] All four men did their best to emphasize the insalubrity of the places they described, linking them to the proliferation of disease and unable to hide their concerns regarding the best and fastest ways to cleanse them.

Preconceptions about insalubrious regions were hardly limited to the African coast, as other tropical regions including Brazil and the Caribbean carved their own individual reputations as injurious sites where Europeans went to find a quick death.[8] Places like Havana and Rio de Janeiro, for example, had their own epidemiological challenges at different times during the nineteenth century; challenges that were reported and discussed across the western hemisphere. In addition to frequent outbreaks of gastrointestinal diseases and smallpox, Havana was the site of recurrent epidemics of yellow fever, dengue fever, and cholera throughout the first half of the century. When Robert Jameson described the conditions in the port in the early 1820s, he echoed almost word for word analogous descriptions given by some of his contemporaries who had described unhygienic African regions, and the indifference shown by those who had managed to stay alive in them:

> The foreign vessels that arrive here suffer greatly. Whole crews are swept off within a few weeks of their arrival, and great difficulty is found in procuring hands for the home passage. . . . Indeed there is scarcely an European who escapes an attack . . . but here, as in the ranks of the battle, the survivors, habituated to the dropping around them, scarcely think of turning to note the victim.[9]

Although Brazil escaped for decades the worst ravages of diseases like cholera and yellow fever, the latter finally arrived to stay in the late 1840s, causing panic and chaos all along the coast, from the Amazonian regions to the
south of Rio de Janeiro.[10] Whereas in Rio de Janeiro, Africans carried on
slave ships were repeatedly blamed for the arrival of yellow fever, in Salvador de Bahia the authorities also made a point of highlighting how the
"overflowing of rivers," the "filth of the city," the "burial of the dead in the
churches," and the "absolute want of a medical police" had contributed to
aggravating the lethal effects of the epidemics.[11] Not even the old recourse of
establishing strict quarantines was enough to keep the dreaded diseases
away.

In Brazil, in Cuba, and along the African coast, the exchanges of peoples, animals, fluids, and merchandises constituted daily occurrences that
could hardly be stopped or controlled, even if authorities on both sides of
the Atlantic fantasized about the best ways of containing rapidly spreading
diseases. Slave-trade contact zones, on land and at sea, were primed morbid
ecosystems where humans fought an uninterrupted battle against diseases
whose causes were often unknown, and where culturally constructed categories of illnesses were shaped and reshaped as health practitioners from
diverse backgrounds came together, turning these deadly spaces into what
historian Katherine Paugh has referred to as "dense site[s] for the exchange
of medical knowledge."[12]

Trading in human beings unavoidably came accompanied by complementary activities that made the business even more hazardous. Likewise,
the efforts to bring the slave trade to an end also included a series of undertakings that were similarly dangerous. To be sure, just as it was the case in
American ports like Havana, Santiago de Cuba, Salvador de Bahia, and Rio
de Janeiro, most of the slave trading spots along the coast of Africa, from the
Senegambia to Benguela, Mozambique, and Quelimane, had long-standing
reputations for being visibly unhealthy.

Likewise, slave vessels were themselves quintessential slave-trade
contact zones, where death and disease were almost perennial residents and
where the lack of ventilation, the heat, and the humidity led at least one
health practitioner to suggest that slave ships themselves were the source of

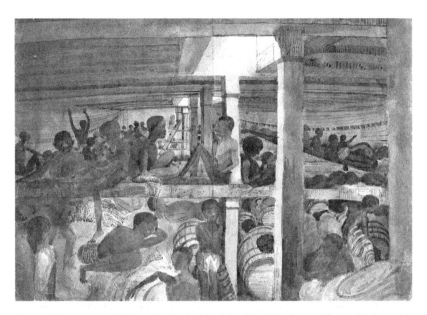

Fig. 2. Recaptured Africans in the hold of the Spanish slaver *Albanoz* in the mid-1840s, according to Lieutenant Francis Meynell. NMM: Personal Collections. Francis Meynell, Mey/2.

a disease such as yellow fever.[13] Examples revealing these unhealthy conditions abounded. For example, when the Portuguese cruiser *Audaz* seized the slave ship *Tâmega* in February 1839 just off Benguela, its sailors were shocked to find a number of dead bodies that had been kept on board by the vessel's crew in a state of complete putrefaction for no apparent reason.[14] On the American side of the Atlantic, these "pestilent" vessels were deemed to be potential carriers of "agents of infection and death," and as such were closely watched by medical, civil, and military authorities, especially in times of epidemics such as those that occurred in Cuba in 1833 and 1852, and in Brazil in the late 1840s.[15]

On slave ships, as in most ports where the slave trade and anti–slave trade activities took place, men, women, and children were exposed not only to likely acts of callousness and negligence but also to poor nutrition, frequently adverse weather conditions, harmful environments, and the diseases that accompanied them. Subjugating both people and environments was a necessary endeavor that required the attention of all those involved with the slave trade in this period. In the particular case of unhealthy environments, this desired subjugation was usually attained through a combination of prophylactic measures and the modification of human behavior.

Contact zones, including those within the nineteenth-century slave trade, were, after all, spaces where "people geographically and historically separated" could meet each other, establishing "ongoing relationships."[16] Within them African, European, and American peoples interacted, exchanging merchandises, ideas, news, body fluids, and diseases. A perhaps unintended result of these exchanges were the narratives of dread and despair produced by those who were separated from their relatives and friends to be sold as slaves, of those who visited and inhabited them as slave dealers, as navy personnel engaged in bringing human trafficking to an end, and as colonial officers and health practitioners of various kinds.

These narratives frequently alluded to gruesome events and inhuman actions, from those involving extreme punishments to even more violent encounters. Central to almost all of them were descriptions and explanations—often hopeless—of the diseases they encountered, of the best ways to prevent their occurrence, and of their effects on the human body and psyche. In Europe and the Americas, those effects were frequently stated and overstated during the period, leading to public and private debates about the epidemiological benefits of continuing the slave trade—in the case of Spaniards, Portuguese, Brazilians—and about the merits and consequences of continuing the efforts to abolish it—in the case of the British and later on the Americans, French, and Portuguese. In sum, actors on both sides of the nineteenth-century slave-trade business—proponents and opponents—continuously contended with the disease environments in which that business took place. As visitors to the slave-trade contact zones were exposed to these diseases, their tragic stories—and on occasion, the tales of the enslaved Africans they trafficked—were told and retold, creating and reproducing fears and anxieties, old and new.

Prophylaxis and prevention were then essential, as the diseases of the transatlantic slave trade were nothing short of obstacles that had to be overcome in order to trade in human beings, and also to "civilize" Africa and to open it for business—and eventually to facilitate a more aggressive type of colonialism. The well-recorded and publicized travels of European explorers like Joseph Richie, Dixon Denham, René Caillié, Hugh Clapperton, the Lander brothers, and all those involved in successive expeditions up the Niger River from the early 1830s onward, demonstrated the challenge presented by diseases to any particular nation or individual willing to engage in trading or colonial endeavors in Africa. In the slave-trade contact zones and beyond, diseases then became not only obstacles but also history-shaping entities.[17]

The Hygienic Challenge

As a deadly epidemic of yellow fever spread across Atlantic Africa in the late 1820s and early 1830s, slave traders, colonial officers, and anti–slave trade personnel struggled to find ways of limiting its destructive effects. In March 1830 Commodore Francis A. Collier, the commander of HMS *Sybille,* one of the Royal Navy ships to be affected by the disease, complained about the mortality on board, noting that even the vessel's assistant surgeon had perished as a result. Collier also reported that the crew had been forced to go under quarantine for fifteen days since its arrival in Saint Helena, bemoaning the lack of effectiveness of "every precaution" taken, including repeated attempts at fumigating and whitewashing the ship. Ultimately, Collier concluded that "the best means of getting rid of the sickness" was sailing "without loss of time, into cooler weather."[18]

The story of HMS *Sybille* as told by Commodore Collier underlines the challenge faced by all those who visited or inhabited the slave-trade contact zones during the first seven decades of the nineteenth century.[19] In addition to having to deal with an already existing disease that was decimating his crew, Collier was just as interested in preventing more disease, and with this in mind, he ordered "every precaution" taken to improve the health aboard. From the outside, the *Sybille* and its crew were compelled to observe a strict quarantine by the British authorities of Saint Helena. Seeing that rather than improving, health on board continued to deteriorate, Commodore Collier took the only sensible choice available to him, determining to sail south toward a more temperate climate, where, eventually, things got better. Like Commodore Collier, many other Atlantic actors of this period were confronted with dangerous and desperate situations that required extreme measures.

This hygienic challenge was equally confronted by slave dealers, slave-ship captains, anti–slave trade patrols, colonial officers, and every other visitor or resident within the slave-trade contact zones. In order to contain these diseases, all relied on their own understanding and interpretations of what diseases they were, how they came into existence, and how they spread and killed. For Europeans and Americans, these containment measures, regardless of their effectiveness, served a double purpose, as they also contributed to defining "racial and sexual identity" throughout the changing Atlantic world of the nineteenth century.[20]

As the slave trade expanded in spite of renewed international efforts to bring it to an end, and as protocolonialist ventures based on trade and gunboat diplomacy became more of a norm, "lines of hygiene" turned into "boundaries of rule," allowing for territorial expansion, subjugation of peoples, and the creation of what Alison Bashford has referred to as "spatial forms of governance."[21] The sanitation of "poisonous" environments, the increasing use of quarantines, and the experimentation in human bodies were all outcomes of a "dream of hygienic containment" that also promoted a colonialist and free-trade agenda intended to benefit those Western governments and traders who were willing to take advantage of the opportunities that Africa offered.

Central to these efforts was the need to reduce morbidity and mortality. While noncontagionist practitioners promoted sanitary measures that targeted the environmental origins of disease, their contagionist colleagues encouraged the implementation of controls and quarantines in order to stop diseases from spreading. Even though their approaches were significantly different, a prevailing "tacit consensus about infection" meant that their suggestions were indistinctly implemented, oftentimes in parallel, throughout the Atlantic world.[22]

There is little doubt that the vast majority of those who visited or inhabited the slave-trade contact zones for most of the period studied here assumed that diseases were a result of a combination of environmental factors and humoral imbalances. Likewise, there is arguably enough evidence to suggest that they often attached a significant weight to human behavior within the contact zones too.

Prevailing miasma theories proposed that epidemic and endemic diseases were the results of unhealthy environments. Swamps, lakes, rivers, rotten wood, heat, and other hazards were all factored into the appearance and transmission of diseases within the slave-trade contact zones.[23] Exposure, especially a prolonged one, to these types of surroundings was often blamed for a wide range of diseases, including the various fevers that affected men, women, and children in the tropical and subtropical regions. The sanitation and curing of these environments—including ships—thus became a priority for all those involved in the slave trade and its abolition throughout the Atlantic. Health practitioners frequently pointed out the dangers associated with these environments and the fundamental need to avoid exposure in order to transform them into healthier settings. James Boyle, for instance, wrote in 1831 about the "noxious effluvia" that pervaded many regions along the Atlantic coast of West Africa. While discussing its characteristics on the Gambia River, he pointed out that these effluvia, in combination with the moisture left after the rain combined with high temperatures to form "the great cause of fever and of ague" that prevailed in the area.[24] In his journal written through 1847, Edward Heath, surgeon of HMS *Rapid,* reflected similar points of view: when some of the vessel's crew had spent five nights being repeatedly bitten by mosquitoes in a mangrove swamp, Heath blamed the considerable number of cases of fever that he diagnosed soon afterward on "exhalations" from the swamp.[25] Years earlier, in the early 1820s, Captain John Adams also attributed the "extreme unhealthiness" on his vessel on the "marsh miasmata and the noxious gas evolved from vegetable matter in a state of decomposition," almost at the same time that a counterpart in the French navy, Ernest de Cornulier, had suggested that "the putrid exhalations from the swamps that surround Senegal" were to blame for the constant presence of "dysentery and pernicious fevers" that prevailed there.[26]

Alongside the presence of miasma and putrefaction, other environmental factors were considered to play important roles in the development

of unhealthy habitats. Tropical rains, sun rays, heat, dews, charged atmospheres, and the like were often linked to the existence of miasma and morbid exhalations, and on occasion were even blamed for producing them. Of
these factors, tropical rains were perhaps the most feared, as the observable
relation between rains and fevers was apparent to all those who inhabited
and visited the slave-trade contact zones.

There was little doubt that tropical rains were considered to be harmful for the European constitutions. For instance, in the Portuguese territories south of the equator, references to the links between tropical rains and
the increase of "poisonous" or "pestilential" exhalations were repeatedly
cited. The Portuguese in Angola even had a name for the rains' effects on
human health: the *carneirada*.[27] In his essay on the diseases of Angola, published in 1799, José Pinto de Azeredo established a clear connection between the rains, the "fermentation of rotten plants," and the subsequent
fevers, or *carneirada,* which affected the local population as soon as the
rains arrived.[28] More than sixty years later, Francisco Travassos Valdez also
made the same connection, referring to the consequences of these rains and
the great fever or *grande carneirada* that followed them.[29]

This noticeable relationship between rain and fevers was also frequently observed on the American side of the Atlantic. In Havana, Robert
Jameson went as far as linking the "direful yellow fever" with the preclusion
of "free circulation of air" and the creation of "stagnant clouds of fetid vapours" that often followed the rains.[30] During a visit of HMS *Serpent* to Port
Royal in 1835, George McLaren also established this link when he wrote in
his diary, "It is the rainy season, and it promises to be an unhealthy one";
already by the time he wrote these lines, yellow fever had sent "many a fine
fellow . . . to the palisades."[31]

The effects of the sun, the heat, and occasionally the dews, were also
recurrently considered to be responsible for the propagation of disease
within the slave-trade contact zones. Their effects on human bodies and the
environment were apparent for all to see. In a report sent to Captain General Mariano Ricafort in 1833, a group of Cuban patricians made it abun-
dantly clear that "the multitude of [African] corpses" found along Cuban
beaches in a state of decomposition due to the sun and heat were "a source

of continuous infection" that had to be prevented by all means possible.[32] On the other side of the Atlantic, a number of British health practitioners echoed each other while pointing out to their superiors the need to avoid by all means unnecessary exposure to these elements. John Bell, the acting surgeon to the forces in the Gambia in 1826, reflected that a combination of "the heat of the sun" during the day and the "heavy dews" at night had led to numerous cases of fever and dysentery among the soldiers garrisoned in this outpost.[33] William Ferguson, Bell's counterpart at Sierra Leone, also cautioned his superiors about the need to guard "against too free exposure to sun, rain, and night dews," while Alexander Stewart, who was also based at Sierra Leone, blamed "the vertical rays of the scorching sun" for the increasing amount of "noxious vapours" and resulting diseases observed at Freetown since he had taken his post there.[34]

Sun, heat, and dews were said to be particularly harmful to the physical constitutions and mental strength of white men. Constantine Keenan, surgeon of HMS *Ranger,* advised in 1861 that white men "should only be exposed to the sun when necessary," and suggested to make a better use of Kroomen—a group of West Africans employed as sailors—during the hours of sun, in order to carry out any heavy work.[35] European and American visitors to the slave-trade contact zones regularly discussed the sun's effects on their own health. That was the case of German traveler and probable slave trader C. H. Van Zütphen, who after carelessly leaving his feet exposed to the sun while reading a book on board the slave ship in which he had traveled to Africa, was burned so badly that he was almost "incapable of walking" for at least two days.[36] In some extreme cases the sun and the heat were even blamed for causing some of the most inexplicable and lethal diseases found in Atlantic Africa. For example, in his book on Sierra Leone, published in 1843, Robert Clarke casually commented that "one of the most common causes" of sleeping sickness, or what he called *lethargus,* was the "exposure to an attack of Coup de Soleil."[37]

Atmospheric changes and variations were also frequently perceived to have significant impact on the health of anyone inhabiting or visiting the slave-trade contact zones. Dénis de Trobriand, the author of one of the few memoirs left by a nineteenth-century slave trader, recalled that in "the vicinity of the autumnal equinox" the "transitions of the atmosphere" were never as complete as they were in Europe, a circumstance that certainly affected the health of any European embarked in a slave-trading expedition.[38] Almost all references to the atmospheres of the slave-trade contact zones included epithets such as *oppressive, harsh,* and *lethal,* and were often linked to the lack of fresh air and appropriate ventilation. Keenan himself was as clear as he could have been when he annotated in his journal that at Fernando Po the atmosphere was usually "still and oppressive" and that in these periods of calm "scarcely a ripple was seen on the surface of the water."[39] Equally, Dr. Young, who had been deployed at the Gold Coast in the first half of the 1820s, referred to the unwholesomeness of the place, which was, in his view, a combination of various factors, including "the moist atmosphere" and the "thick jungle," which impeded "a thorough ventilation."[40]

Effluvia, miasma, and poisonous emanations were all perceived as agents of contamination of the atmosphere, capable of turning perfectly breathable air into a toxic and potentially deadly "inhalable stench."[41] Sea breezes, on the other hand, were considered to be the most readily available and effective remedy against these unhealthy environments. Sending feverish patients out to sea for a few days, and locating slave-trading factories and anti–slave trade outposts in places where the sea breezes blew, became common practice whenever possible. Following this logic, in 1831 Sierra Leone Governor Alexander Findlay blamed "the thick underwood and trees" surrounding Freetown for intercepting the sea breeze, consequently rendering "the town unhealthy."[42] That sea winds were held in high esteem was confirmed by renowned traveler Richard Burton during his visit to the Gambia in the late 1850s, when he commented that in those lands the locals referred to the ocean breeze as "the Doctor," due to its healing powers.[43]

In addition to theories related to the impact upon human health of environmental and meteorological factors such as the rain, sun rays, the heat, and dews were other less popular opinions. The French physician Mathieu Audouard considered slave ships themselves to be the source of epidemics of yellow fever.[44] According to Audouard, yellow fever was a product of the appalling conditions found in the hold of slave vessels, and the climates that were usually associated with its origin were merely of a secondary nature.[45] Although Audouard's theory was almost universally rejected, it was at times evaluated and discussed throughout the Atlantic world, having a final moment of revival in Brazil, when yellow fever turned into a serious health emergency in the late 1840s and early 1850s.[46]

Ultimately, when focusing on the potentially lethal qualities of any particular environments, actors throughout the various slave-trade contact zones were presented with a wide array of measures that could be taken in order to reduce the morbidity associated with these spaces. Sanitizing and, if possible, curing these spaces—from urban centers and slave-trading factories to vessels used either for the slave trade or for its eradication—became a central activity for anyone with the power and capabilities to do so.

The nineteenth century thus was a time of renewed focus on the sanitation of unhealthy environments, which coincided with the peak of miasma theory. Sanitizing and curing slave-trade contact zones was an integral part of the often-ineffective policies of hygienic containment considered necessary to allow Europeans and Americans to survive the diseases associated with these environments and, eventually, to subjugate their peoples. These needs were frequently expressed through instructions about finding low-morbidity "dry and cool" places where new settlements could be started, and where ailing patients could be taken care of.[47] Granted, this was not always possible, especially in the case of the African slave-trade contact zones, as Commodore Matthew C. Perry of the U.S. anti–slave trade African squadron pointed out in 1844. In a missive sent to the secretary of the navy, Perry commented that in his experience there was no place in West Africa "from the Cambia [sic] to the Equator where the annual mortality of unacclimated white persons living on shore would not be, in the present uncleared state of the country, from 30 to 50 per cent of the whole number."[48] In this letter Commodore Perry also ardently emphasized that high mortality due to tropical diseases not only affected human beings but also killed cattle and other animals, rendering them useless for consumption even if they survived.[49]

Although most of the concrete work of sanitation was carried out in the actual slave-trade contact zones, a number of initiatives were thought of and put into practice by Europeans and Americans even before they embarked on their outward journeys. The instructions given by slave-ship owners to their captains before sailing for the coast of Africa demonstrate that cleanliness and sanitation aboard slave vessels were considered to be fundamental for the prevention of disease among the human cargo and their traders. Similar directives during this period by anti–slave trade patrol commanders before sailing for Africa point to a parallel attention to detail about sanitation among those who aspired to stop slave traders. Perhaps the best-known mechanism of this objective was the ventilation machine commissioned by the British from David Boswell Reid and subsequently fitted on the vessels built for the Niger Expedition in 1841.[50] These ships, according to Howard Temperley, were provided with "fanners, which could be driven by the engines when the ships were in motion or by the action of the river currents on the paddles when they were moored."[51]

The new ventilation methods employed in the struggle against so-called rarified atmospheres led to new important measures, which were taken in order to improve the health of those inhabiting or visiting the slave-trade contact zones. Along the African coast and virtually in every main destination for the illegal slave trade in the Americas after 1820, precautions were taken in order to provide a better quality of air or to protect those who were exposed to any injurious atmospheres from its possible effects.

In places as diverse as Freetown, Havana, and Salvador de Bahia, orders were issued to clean the streets and to situate those who were affected by contagious diseases outside urban perimeters.[52] On ships of all kinds similar measures were taken. For example, in 1861, Constantine Keenan, aware of the need to take prophylactic measures to improve the health of the crew of HMS *Ranger,* ordered that the awnings of the vessel should be well locked at night, while Alexander Bryson proposed in 1847 to use air pumps to keep the ships ventilated at all times.[53]

Ship commanders of the anti–slave trade squadrons were among the first to take measures to improve the quality of the air breathed by the crews and the Africans seized on board slave ships alongside their captors. For example, in the summer of 1860, Captain Thomas Dornin, commander of USS *San Jacinto,* was keen to stress how he and his officers had endeavored to provide "as much fresh air as possible" to the 619 Africans they had

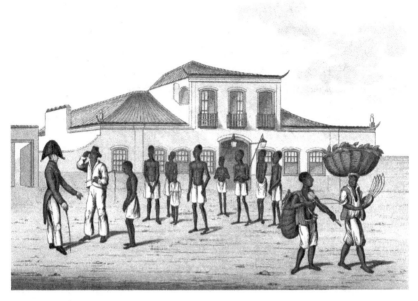

Fig. 3. Recently arrived Africans taken out to breathe fresh air in in Rio de Janeiro, c. 1819–20. Henry Chamberlain, *Views and costumes of the city and neighborhood of Rio de Janeiro, Brazil, from drawings taken by Lieutenant Chamberlain, Royal Artillery, during the years 1819 and 1820, with descriptive explanations* (London: McLean, 1822).

taken days before from a slaver.[54] Likewise, in March 1841, the Anglo-Brazilian Mixed Commission court judges at Rio de Janeiro agreed on a series of provisions to be offered to a group of recently captured Africans, which included moving them to HMS *Crescent,* where they could be relieved of the deadly air they were sharing in the hold of the slave ship where they have been kept till then.[55]

Fumigation, disinfestation, whitewashing, and other cleansing schemes also became, to "an almost fanatical" level, common practice during the period, especially on vessels involved in one way or another with the slave trade.[56] There were repeated discussions about the most efficient methods and products to disinfest decks and holds. Spraying vinegar was one of the most frequently used procedures, probably due to the easy availability of the product. Examples of the use of vinegar for disinfestation purposes are numerous. A case in question was that of the commander of the Portuguese anti–slave trade squadron, Francisco António Gonçalves Cardoso, who in 1849 noted in the journal of the ship under his command, the *Mondego,* that he had taken "all the hygienic measures, such as spreading perfumes on deck, and squirting vinegar," in order to keep the ship as clean as possible.[57]

Vinegar seems to have been a disinfectant of choice, not just because it was easy to find and apply but also because it could be used for multiple purposes, including cooking.[58] Some health practitioners during the period, however, such as Alexander Bryson, were skeptical about its real efficacy in purifying morbid environments. In 1847 Bryson stated that although vinegar was useful for covering "the odour arising from the bodies of the sick, or from the decomposing matters in the hold," it was still largely ineffective when it came to "staying the march of disease."[59]

Rather than relying on vinegar, or even on the also popular chloride of lime, which was said to be as foul smelling as bilge water, Bryson suggested the heat of burning charcoal as a much more successful disinfectant; even better, he recommended the use of chloride of zinc:

> By numerous experiments performed in various vessels in different parts of the world . . . it appears that the instant the slime or rubbish in the limbers of a ship becomes saturated with a solution of the salt, the process of decomposition–putrid fermentation, is instantly arrested, and consequently also the liberation of mephitic gases.[60]

Other products used for the fumigation of slave-trade contact zones during this period, both on land and at sea, were nitric acid, common salt, and a mildly antiseptic mixture of calcium hydroxide and chalk, regularly used to whitewash buildings, vessels, and nearly any kind of standing structure.[61]

From a prophylactic viewpoint, these measures had only a limited effect, as they frequently failed to address the real causes of the diseases they were targeting. However, the strategies of burning vegetable matter, drying swamps and pools where mosquitoes bred, whitewashing walls, and keeping ships in a state of cleanliness may have combined to limit the ravages of disease among those inhabiting and visiting the slave-trade contact zones. Frequent fumigation and disinfestation in particular may have eliminated, even if serendipitously, a number of disease-carrying vectors like mosquitoes, ticks, and cockroaches.

As a final resort, and when confronted with the failure of all measures to transform environments, seamen, traders, and officials in the slave-trade contact zones attempted on occasion to relocate from particularly morbid and deadly sites to other locations that were considered to be healthier. To be sure, these attempts were not easily undertaken. Although for some slave traders along the African coast, moving from one place to another was not unheard of, when it came to larger urban centers, an enterprise of such magnitude was fraught with all sorts of problems.

The prominent case of Sierra Leone was especially complicated. The colony already had a growing reputation as a white man's grave by the late 1820s, and British authorities began to consider the very real possibility of repositioning it, including the Liberated African Department, elsewhere along the African coast. By 1829, the isles of Los, for example, had been proposed as a much healthier environment.[62] Next the British seriously considered the possibility of moving to Port Clarence, in Fernando Po, a territory that had been leased from the Spanish in 1827.[63] News about the possible relocation of the British began to circulate in late 1827, and already in May 1828 it was widely believed that Fernando Po was the most likely and desirable destination for such a project.[64] By then Captain William Owen had been put in charge of Fernando Po as a governor, with the goal of turning the island into the future base of "the Britannic forces along the coast of West Africa."[65] Ultimately, when the yellow fever epidemic of 1829–30 reached Fernando Po, the idea of relocating the British colony was abandoned, as the island proved to be just as hazardous to the health of Europeans and Africans alike as Sierra Leone had been.[66]

Environment-based approaches to address the hygienic challenge presented to all those inhabiting and visiting the slave-trade contact zones were habitually combined with various levels and types of regulations to human behavior. Just as the environment needed to be sanitized and controlled, so did human behavior. Abiding by socially acceptable norms of

behavior considered to be "civilized"—as opposed to the conduct and com-
portment of Africans and other non-Western peoples—constituted a vital
guidance for anyone hoping to survive the tropical diseases associated with
the slave-trade contact zones. These instructions, however, were mostly di-
rected to European and American visitors and inhabitants, as "uncivilized"
Africans in particular were considered to be "less liable to disease than civilized persons."[67]

A number of moral considerations, including the need for a frugal life,
abstinence from sex, and temperance, were deemed necessary for those willing to turn to a career as a slave trader on land or at sea, as well as for those
attached to the various anti–slave trade squadrons, and Western settlements
along the coasts of West, West Central, and East Africa. A strong Christian
religious sentiment underpinning these moral considerations resulted in advice and prohibitions against drinking alcohol, indulging in gluttony, having
sexual relations, exposing bodies to the elements, and interacting with the
locals more than necessary. Of course, the inhabitants and visitors to the
slave-trade contact zones did all the things they were advised against, and
many lived long lives in Africa in spite of their distempered behavior.

Notable among them were navy personnel and soldiers from the various nations involved in the patrolling against the slave trade, as well as slave
factors and slave-trade ship crews. Temperance and abstinence were perhaps the topics more frequently discussed by those trying to establish a direct relationship between human behavior and the chances of being attacked
by a disease. Community moral arbiters, like religious missionaries, colonial governors and officers, slave-ship owners, and navy commanders, all
called repeatedly for the men under their orders to stay away from spirits as
much as possible.

Throughout the first half of the century, temperance was a topic of
discussion across Europe and the Americas. These discussions even led to
the rise of a temperance movement in the British Isles and other parts of the
Atlantic, and influenced the ways in which Europeans, Americans, and Africans interacted with one another throughout the Atlantic world.[68] Some
of the main authors related to this movement used on occasion the texts
produced by health practitioners and missionaries who had been in direct

contact with the diseases associated with the slave trade. William Benjamin
Carpenter, for example, relied heavily on the narratives of Dr. William Daniell and Reverend Charles Rattray while reviewing the effects of alcohol
upon European constitutions in the tropical regions.[69]

Some of the most important authors to discuss slave-trade diseases
during the period were keen to stress the need for temperance for all those
who were to come into contact with the slave-trade contact zones. Robert
Clarke, after spending eighteen years in Sierra Leone, felt his duty to note, in
poetic undertones and referencing the need for a temperate life, "If nature
wears a perpetual smile in this quarter of the world, it is to those only who
listen to her teachings."[70] Peter Leonard was also emphatic when he wrote in
the early 1830s that "temperance in this climate [West Africa] is imperatively
necessary." Nonetheless, Leonard, like Daniell and Carpenter years later, did
not recommend absolute abstinence from alcoholic beverages, considering it
to be just as injurious as excessive consumption.[71] Other authors, such as
Bryson, were keen to highlight the extent of the temperate challenge by pointing out the ease of access to alcoholic beverages along the African shores:

> There is no part of the station, no tribe, however rude and prim-
> itive, that have not at hand some species of intoxicating liquor,
> ready to offer to the men for a small remuneration, the instant
> they set their foot on shore. Trade rum of the worst description
> at the Gambia, Sierra Leone, and on the Gold Coast, aqua ardi-
> ente at Bissao, Princes' Island, and the Island of St. Thomas;
> and palm wine in every creek and river where there are palm
> trees in the bush, and natives resident on the shore.[72]

Not surprisingly, then, blaming the occurrence of disease on the drunken
behavior of Africans, soldiers, sailors, and settlers was common. A. Nicholl,
for example, blamed the swollen bills of mortality of Sierra Leone in 1820 on
the "adventurers, seafaring people and by those Spaniards that are brought
here by the HMS ships of war in captured slave vessels."[73] More than twenty
years later, Augustus P. Arkwright made clear in a letter to his mother that in
Sierra Leone, even though complaints about the climate were continual,

only "those who care for nothing" suffered from it.[74] William Ferguson also pointed out in the mid-1820s that he believed it impossible to determine the real causes of disease among British soldiers in Sierra Leone, as the "very dissolute lives" they led made it difficult to "afford the surest criterion for judging the influence of the climate on European constitutions."[75]

On the other side of the ocean, similar theories prevailed. In Brazil, for example, John Candler and Wilson Burgess blamed sailors' "reckless manner of life" and "determined drinking habits" for their vulnerability to "whatever epidemic may prevail."[76] Several visitors to Cuba during the period also found the behavior of a random assortment of people, including African slaves, Catalonian traders, and foreign sailors in the busy port of Havana responsible for the disappearance of good manners and for the increase of epidemic diseases.[77]

A variety of measures were taken by various Atlantic actors to address the abuse of alcohol. Richard Reece, for example, produced a *Medical Guide for Tropical Climates,* in which he emphasized, among many other proposals, the abstinence from alcoholic drinks.[78] In the U.S. Navy, Lieutenant Andrew Hull Foote ruled his African squadron ship with "strong religious and reforming views," among which the total abstinence from consuming alcohol was essential.[79] In Sierra Leone, by the end of the 1820s, Acting Governor Henry John Ricketts, went so far as to recommending to the secretary of the Church Missionary Society that "suitable provisions should be made for watching over the morals of the old settlers in the mountain villages," an order presumably aimed at policing any abuses of both alcohol consumption and sexual relations among the populations of these villages.[80]

Living an honorable life also meant refraining from extramarital sexual encounters in the slave-trade contact zones. These encounters did indeed lead to the spread of sexually transmitted diseases.[81] Cautions against drinking alcohol were frequently accompanied by similar warnings against the "passions" of sexual excesses.[82] With that in mind, slave traders, anti-slave trade ship commanders, and authorities throughout the Atlantic repeatedly tried to keep men separated from women. That was the case in many if not most slave vessels during the period, and often in reception centers like those in Sierra Leone and Saint Helena.[83]

Notoriously, some slave traders on land and at sea had well-documented sexual relations with African women. These relations were often coerced and violent. John Ormond Jr., Pedro Blanco, and Francisco Félix de Souza were said to have harems or seraglios near their factories on the rivers Pongo, Gallinas, and Ouidah.[84] Others like slave-ship captains Antonio José Puga and Alvaro Correia de Morais, were revealed to have been taking advantage of their positions to abuse some of the enslaved women they had acquired in Africa. Puga referred to the sixth commandment in a letter to John González, noticing that he "had been so fortunate as to have had four virgins brought" to him for sexual purposes the moment he had arrived at Pablo Álvarez Simidel's factory in Gallinas in 1838.[85] Likewise, Correia de Morais was praised by a fellow slave trader in sexually charged undertones, for having the opportunity of getting to choose the "naked black women" he wanted for himself.[86] At a more generic level, sexual violence against women could be manifested in other ways. For example, during this period, there were rumors that suggested that slave dealers along the coast of Africa would force African women to take potions "to suppress the menstrual flow" just before they were embarked on their ships.[87]

At sea, the situation was often at its worst. Several vessels' crews during this period were accused of violence against the enslaved women carried to the Americas in the holds and decks of their ships. Particularly distressing were the stories pertaining to the Portuguese schooner *Arrogante* in 1837 and the Spanish schooner *Jesus Maria* in 1841. In both cases, reports abounded of rapes preceded and followed by beatings. In some instances, sailors were accused of murdering African women who refused to have sexual relations with them. A woman called Yacca, for example, was beaten, murdered, and thrown overboard when she rejected one of the *Arrogante*'s sailors, and another woman was killed on the *Jesus Maria*.[88] In the latter case, the captain, Vicente Morales, and the crew were accused of having raped and killed children as well.[89]

British personnel detached to the anti–slave trade squadron were also accused of all kind of excesses, including those of the flesh.[90] In the mid-1830s, when the hulk of HMS *Conflict* was destined to receive the crews arriving in Sierra Leone on board prize vessels, there were rumors

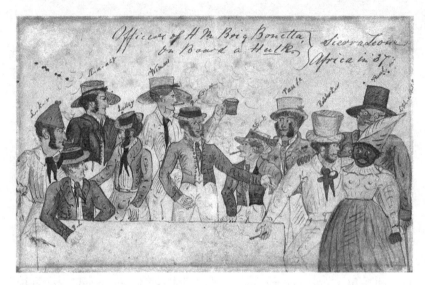

Fig. 4. HMS *Bonetta*'s sailors on board of a hulk, almost certainly HMS *Conflict*, in Sierra Leone, 1837. NMM: ZBA4579.

about the irregular conduct of many of the officers and sailors who were sent there to wait for their respective vessels to catch up with them in the British West African outpost. This sort of behavior was recorded in a watercolor from 1837, in which the officers and sailors of HMS *Bonetta* were depicted engaging in smoking, drinking, and carnal activities, in the latter case with an African woman.[91] In Havana, around the same dates, the soldiers attached to HMS *Romney* were accused at times of landing in Havana and of developing relationships with women in the neighborhood of Casablanca, where the vessel was moored.[92]

Other than temperance and sexual restraint, eating wholesome foods and dressing appropriately were believed to be the best approaches to staying healthy in the slave-trade contact zones. Almost every medical guide or manual devoted to the best ways of surviving and living in the so-called torrid zones had plenty of recommendations, such as boiling water before drinking it, eating moderately, and sleeping in spaces where breezes could carry away insects.[93] In the "System of Medical Conduct for European in Tropical Climates" included in his book published in 1814, Richard Reece proposed,

among other things, that readers drink only boiled water, eat plenty of vege-
tables, take cold baths in the mornings and before dinner, wear cotton clothes,
and do exercise only "of the passive kind."[94] James Ormiston McWilliam
gave a series of similar imperatives decades later, including staying dry, taking
baths of lemon juice or rum, drinking coffee before going on duty, exercising,
avoiding water that had not been boiled, eating a healthy diet, drinking wine
and taking quinine according to medical advice.[95] In a similar vein, Robert
Clarke, after being reassigned to the Gold Coast in the late 1850s, commented
on the eating and drinking excesses he had observed in his new destination,
noticing the effects that such behavior had upon human health:

> In my opinion a very great deal of the suffering and disease so
> constantly met with in this climate is occasioned as elsewhere
> by overfeeding which as well as overdrinking has consigned its
> victims to the grave yards of these settlements. Sobriety as re-
> gards eating being quite as necessary to preserve health as tem-
> perance in drinking.[96]

All those involved in the slave-trade contact zones—slave traders, colonial
officers, and anti–slave trade personnel—attempted to contain diseases by
adopting various hygienic practices. These practices, in turn, were derived
from their own understanding of these diseases and the way they were
spread, and depended on the priorities of those carrying out their slave-
trading or anti–slave trade activities. Environment-based approaches to addressing the hygienic challenge were combined with various regulations of
human behavior, which were almost always based on moral considerations.
Ultimately, efforts to contain disease were more often than not politically
tainted and ineffective, at least from the epidemiological point of view.

Bills of Health, Quarantines, and Protocolonial Expansionism

While discussing the value of the bills of health issued by the authorities
in Rio de Janeiro in 1828, a Brazilian bureaucrat went to great lengths to
underline the relationship that had traditionally existed between medicine

and government. In his words, "the alliance of medicine and politics is almost as ancient as these sciences themselves."[97] Bills of health, issued by
authorities all across the Atlantic to vessels departing their ports, were indeed nothing short of political weapons that could facilitate or limit the
movement of peoples and products. In more than one way they constituted
the first line of defense in many of the hygienic containment attempts implemented in the slave-trade contact zones after abolition policies began to affect the ways in which human trafficking was carried out.

For vessels involved in the transatlantic slave trade, bills of health
were a necessary expense that allowed for more effective and successful
transactions and exchanges. These bills of health were part of the papers
confiscated from virtually every vessel seized by anti–slave trade patrols in
the Atlantic after 1820.[98] They were usually certified by local authorities in
ports like Havana, Salvador de Bahia, Luanda, or Cádiz, and frequently en-
dorsed by the consuls of those nations that were involved in the illegal trafficking of Africans.[99] At times and in the hope of appearing more convincing
upon inspection at sea or in their ports of destination, some ships carried
with them two or more bills of health issued by different authorities in different ports at different times.[100] In spite of these extra efforts, however, and
as Jaime Rodrigues has pointed out, they were nothing short of "a formal-
ity" that was "very easy to elude by slave traders."[101] The many reports of
slave vessels that left Africa with clean bills of health but arrived at their
destinations suffering of high morbidity and mortality levels suggest that
these documents were regularly manipulated by slave dealers to fit their
purposes.[102]

More to the point, many of the illegal factories situated alongside the
coast of Africa did not issue bills of health, a circumstance that rendered
those documents obtained upon sailing for Africa inadequate at best, and
almost useless in most cases, as they were unable to account for any health
changes that could have taken place during the time they had spent visiting
African ports.

Equally, from the early years of the nineteenth century, and just as the
slave trade began to come under threat, quarantines became a more frequent hygienic measure to regulate public health and to contain the spread

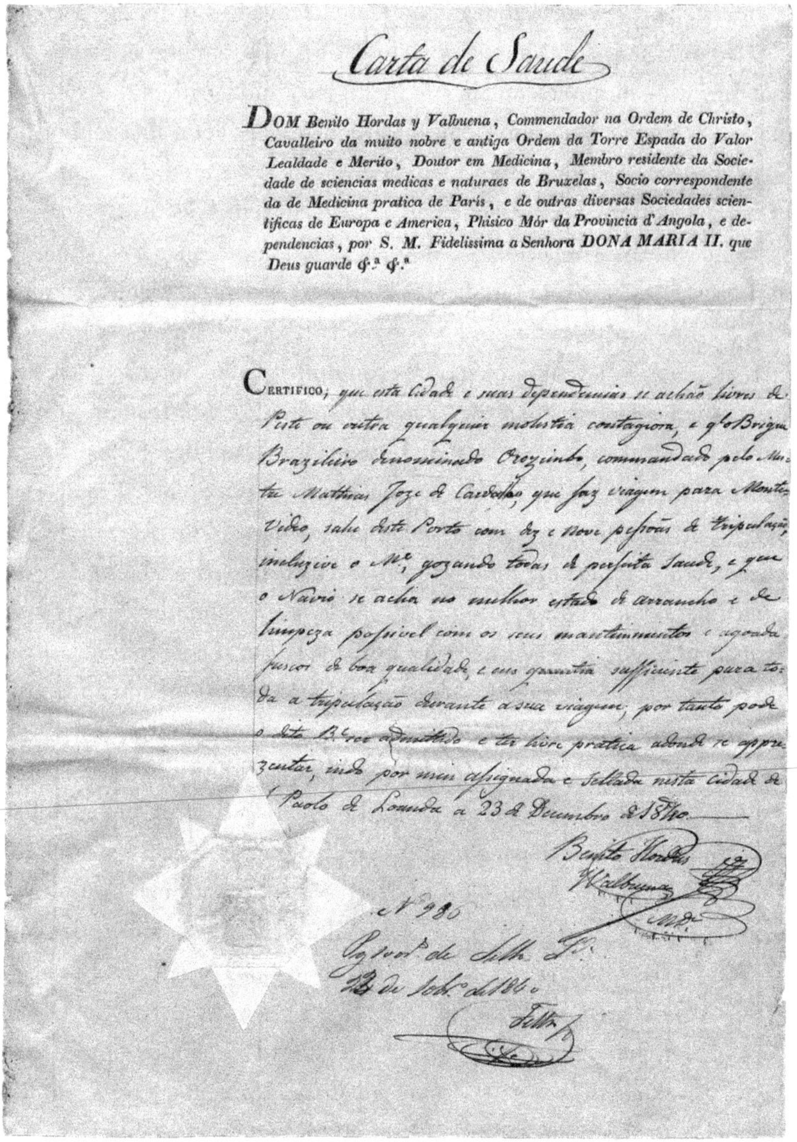

Carta de Saude

DOM *Benito Hordas y Valbuena*, *Commendador na Ordem de Christo*, *Cavalleiro da muito nobre e antiga Ordem da Torre Espada do Valor Lealdade e Merito*, *Doutor em Medicina*, *Membro residente da Socie-dade de sciencias medicas e naturaes de Bruxelas*, *Socio correspondente da de Medicina pratica de Paris*, *e de outras diversas Sociedades scien-tificas de Europa e America*, *Phisico Mór da Provincia d'Angola*, *e de-pendencias*, *por S. M. Fidelissima a Senhora* **DONA MARIA II.** *que Deus guarde &.ª &.ª*

CERTIFICO, que esta Cidade e suas dependencias se achão livres de Peste ou outra qualquer molestia contagiosa, e q'o Brigue Brazileiro denominado Orozimbo, commandado pelo Mestre Mathias Joze de Cardoso, que faz viagem para Monte-video, sahe deste Porto com dez e nove pessoas de tripulação, inclusive o M.e; gozando todas de perfeita Saude, e que o Navio se acha no melhor estado de arrancho e de limpeza possivel com os seus mantimentos e agoada pescados de boa qualidade, e em quantia sufficiente para to-da a tripulação durante a sua viagem; por tanto pode o dito Barco admittido e ter livre pratica aonde se apre-zentar, indo por mim assignado e sellada nesta Cidade de S. Paolo de Loanda a 23 de Dezembro de 1840.——

Benito Hordas
Valbuena
M.e

N 980

Fig. 5. Bill of health, Brazilian brig *Orozimbo*, December, 1840. TNA: Foreign Office, 315/50.

of infectious diseases. Although the real effectiveness of quarantines depended on a series of factors that included the nature of the actual disease
that they were meant to contain and the rigidity and length of the isolation,
they were considered among the best courses of action that authorities
across the Atlantic could implement in order to at least give the impression
of being in control while dealing with potentially lethal diseases.

Like the bills of health, quarantines served both hygienic and political
purposes, as their execution often bestowed those who implemented them
with a rational justification to keep enemies and undesirables at bay. Numerous scholars have pointed out the multiplicity of reasons behind quarantines and the effects that they had on European colonialism, especially
during the nineteenth century.[103] In the words of Alison Bashford, throughout the nineteenth century quarantine stations "multiplied across every
large body of water."[104] This was especially the case in the Atlantic world,
where human trafficking, now carried out illegally, led to the unchecked
dissemination of deadly and debilitating diseases. Quarantine stations were
permanent features in almost every port related to the slave trade. They
were usually situated outside the perimeters of urban centers, on nearby
islands, or at sea, on vessels specifically modified for this purpose.

In Sierra Leone, where thousands of recaptured Africans were landed
throughout the first seven decades of the nineteenth century, the British
used a number of locations to quarantine new arrivals. These included the
town of Wilberforce, to the west of Freetown, where at times there was a
hospital expressly intended to receive smallpox patients; a walled lazaretto
specifically destined to contain potentially contagious patients in the village
of Kissy; and occasional vessels moored in the river just off Kissy.[105] In Havana, quarantine stations to the west of the city had functioned since at least
the late seventeenth century and were still in use during the 1860s.[106] In Rio
de Janeiro, the Casa de Correção was used throughout the period, as were
two vessels, the *Nova Piedade* and the *Crescent.*[107]

The logistics of quarantines in the slave-trade contact zones had its
own peculiar challenges. Whereas quarantines elsewhere, especially in Europe, were normally associated with goods and merchandise, in the Atlantic
they were mostly conceived as ways of regulating human movement.[108] For

those in charge of containing epidemics on both sides of the Atlantic, the distinction between legal and illegal commerce was paramount to the ways in which they executed quarantine measures. In Havana, for example, as a lethal cholera epidemic caused havoc in 1833, medical practitioners and the general public begged the newly appointed captain general to implement a rigorous quarantine, especially targeting vessels arriving from Africa. Petitioners frantically claimed: "If for the licit commerce we have rigorous quarantines, what should not we do with an illicit traffic that threatens our lives and our prosperity?"[109] Although such a despairing request was undoubtedly affected by an extraordinary situation that threatened their lives and fortunes, in reality Cubans had been calling for stronger measures to monitor the slave trade at least since 1820, when two neighbors of Matanzas wrote to Captain General Juan Manuel Cajigal complaining about the lack of controls around the introduction of African men, women, and children onto the island, warning him about the "hazards that these landings . . . could cause to the health, wellness and security of the persons of this neighborhood."[110]

There is little doubt that these requests were listened to and eventually acted upon. Years later, in 1836, Captain General Miguel Tacón informed the British Mixed Commission judges in Havana that all vessels arriving in the port without bills of health, as well as all those that had come into contact with such ships, were being immediately placed on observational quarantines, with the intention of avoiding the spread of new epidemics in the city.[111] The measures discussed by Tacón were in reality much stricter than what he represented in this missive, since the Havana Junta Superior de Sanidad had in fact decided that even ships arriving with a bill of health, but missing a certificate from the Spanish consul at their port of departure, were to be subjected to a period of quarantine of no less than seven days.[112]

Complaints about the institution and effectiveness of quarantines across the Atlantic during this period were abundant. In Saint Helena, George McHenry lamented in 1843 the relaxed nature of quarantine controls within the island, which in his opinion had, within a three-year period, led to the introduction of smallpox seven times from seven different slave ships, "each with numerous patients, labouring under that disease."[113] After observing the situation of the quarantine station at Madeira during a short stop at the island in the late 1850s, Richard Burton also questioned the quarantine measures in place, calling them "arbitrary and exclusive" and commenting that the lazaretto where they were implemented was "wholly neglected."[114]

In fact, the efficacy of these quarantine stations was in itself a source of debate throughout the Atlantic world. Dale Graden has established that in Rio de Janeiro quarantines had been in place a long time before yellow fever arrived in the late 1840s and that they had done little to stop the epidemic from spreading in the city and into other parts of the country.[115] Adrián López Denis and Enrique Beldarraín Chaple have also emphasized that measures taken by the Cuban authorities in the wake of the first and second cholera epidemics of the nineteenth century in 1833 and 1852 did little to contain the spread of the disease, especially as political and commercial interests limited their effectiveness each time.[116]

Strict enforcement and policing of quarantines thus seem likely to have been more about reassuring the public that it was safe than about actually safeguarding public health. Moreover, violations of quarantine regulations occurred virtually everywhere they were established. Sometimes these violations had the tacit consent of local authorities, as, for example, in Saint Helena in 1843, when McHenry criticized the laxity of the island's authorities in enforcing their own orders. A case in question was recorded in May 1826, when the commanding officer of HMS *Maidstone* infringed the quarantine regulations in place at Sierra Leone, where he and his vessel had arrived after seizing a ship full of Africans suffering from smallpox.[117] Among the stern orders he was given—which he was unable to follow to the letter—were to keep a yellow flag constantly hoisted, to avoid any communication with the shore, and to keep at a distance any boats that approached the vessel.[118] In their West African outposts the French had also established severe quarantine measures from the first decades of the century. In Gorée, for example, they had regulations in place for a health practitioner to board every vessel, and they kept a warship in the port to enforced the rules.[119] In Madeira, according to Burton, whenever fevers were "supposed to be on the West Afri-

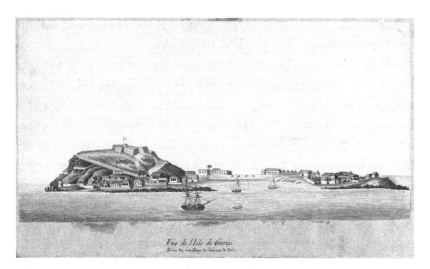

Fig. 6. View of the island of Gorée, c. 1822–23. NMM: LOG/F/4.

can Coast," the Portuguese too would force anyone wanting to land to spend time in their quarantine station, bills of health being "of no avail."[120]

Equally important to legitimizing the validity and efficacy of quarantine policies were the periods of containment and the rules to follow before releasing those who had been confined. Quarantines would regularly last for periods of between five and ten days. Circumstances as diverse as seasons, environments, and health conditions of those to be quarantined could affect the length of time to which vessels, crews, passengers, and trafficked people were subjected. Establishing the appropriate period of time, given the characteristics of each specific disease, could convince the public that the possible spread of the disease was under control. More significant, determining the required measures to be taken ahead of the release of those in quarantine was also essential, as the suspicion that potentially sick people were being released into urban and rural spaces could undermine trust in the general population.

With this in mind, rigorous periods of quarantine were almost always followed by hygienic measures devised to cleanse those who had been confined, as well as the spaces that had confined them. In Sierra Leone after recaptured Africans, slave-trade ship crews, and navy personnel were released from quarantine, the places where they had been kept were regularly fumigated and whitewashed and their clothes destroyed. In 1826, for example, the Africans seized on the Spanish schooner *Iberia* were discharged from their quarters at Wilberforce, but not before their clothes and blankets were destroyed. After their departure, it was also advised that the buildings that had hosted them should be immediately whitewashed.[121] Almost two decades later, in 1844, after the recaptured Africans of the *Aventura* were set free from their quarantine confinement aboard the ship, orders of fumigating and purifying their quarters were issued, also with immediate effect.[122]

Quarantines in the slave-trade contact zones differed in one other important way from quarantines elsewhere. Beyond the obvious fact that they were aimed mostly at controlling human movement, they were also implemented mostly on one side of the slave-trade contact zones, namely the legal side. To date there is no evidence that slave factors engaged in illegal human trafficking along the coasts of West, West Central, and East Africa ever implemented quarantines of any sort. This absence of evidence is not surprising, as quarantines disrupted the trade in human beings and merchandise, and as a result were considered to be detrimental for any lucrative business.

Within the legal realm, however, whenever quarantines were applied and scrupulously enforced, they also acted as a preventive measure to limit the scale of the introduction of Africans into their prearranged destinations in the Americas.[123] But rigorous quarantines also had an effect on the work of Mixed Commission and Vice-Admiralty courts, as they constituted obstacles that blocked the access of abolitionist personnel to the Africans and slave-trade crews that were to be brought before the courts. When the Spanish schooner *Diligencia* was seized in 1835 and taken to Havana with 120 sick Africans on board, the officers of the Mixed Commission court were unable to begin their work, as the vessel was immediately placed in quarantine by the Spanish authorities.[124] Something similar occurred during the adjudications of the brig *Perpetuo Defensor* and the schooner *Aventura* in 1826 and 1844, respectively, when the court officers at Freetown were unable to gain access to and process the ships until the periods of quarantine for each had been met, both having been infected with numerous cases of smallpox.[125]

In the slave-trade contact zones of the nineteenth century, then, both bills of health and quarantines played two main roles. On the one hand, in line with contagionist ideas, they were expected to help contain the spread of disease by providing methods of control and secluded spaces where sick peoples or those who had been exposed to disease could be isolated, observed, and treated. On the other, they functioned as public spectacles, aimed at legitimizing a dream of hygienic containment. As diseases took over vessels and urban and rural settings, every effort was made to fight diseases with these ultimate prophylactic measures, turning them into important components of emerging new Atlantic medical cultures. In the process, those in charge of implementing and policing them also gained an upper hand in the regulation and control of trade, and were given an unexpected boost in their efforts to create and expand their colonial agendas.

On July 15, 1846, Commander Francisco António Gonçalves Cardoso, who had been attached to the Portuguese West African squadron since 1844, wrote to Manoel de Vasconcelos e Pereira de Mello, Baron of Lazarim and major general of the Portuguese Armada, complaining about the high morbidity and mortality faced by his men and by all those assigned to patrol the waters along the coast of Africa in search for slavers. As in many other opportunities, Gonçalves Cardoso lamented that irrespective of the preventative measures taken, his men continued to fall sick; the climate of the regions they were in charge of policing, he noticed, had "the property of diminishing considerably the duration of the personnel" under his orders.[126]

Gonçalves Cardoso's predicament was hardly unique. All those in command of vessels and settlements, regardless of their involvement with the slave trade or its abolition, were confronted with the same pressing needs to prevent disease by all means possible, and they all shared the same frustrations with regard to the limitations of the methods available to them. Gonçalves Cardoso himself was eventually forced to leave his post in 1849 after falling sick, probably of hepatitis. In one of his final missives to Lisbon, he noted that this was the first time in his life he had asked for a leave of absence, and bemoaned that "five years of Africa, not spent with crossed arms, could put out of action even the most robust Alcydes."[127]

In truth, the hygienic challenge presented to this assortment of peoples was immense. In order to reassert their claims to geopolitical spaces,
slave dealers and anti–slave trade forces, including colonists and represen-
tatives of different governments, did everything in their power to increase
the time that their personnel could last in these regions, and to do so in at
least acceptable health. A variety of hygienic measures were taken in the
hope of lessening the morbid and mortal effects of endemic and epidemic
diseases. Central to many of these efforts in the post-1820 Atlantic world
were sanitizing environments, controlling people's movement and behaviors, and implementing quarantines, strategies designed both to keep diseases away and to consolidate protocolonial claims to lands and peoples.

The measures adopted to prevent and contain disease were not always based on reason and observation, although on occasion they followed
the recommendations given by a number of health practitioners in the manuals and guidelines published during this period. Nevertheless, although it
would be nearly impossible to prove it, there are strong grounds to believe
that some of these measures did have some impact in limiting the ravages of
disease. The clearing and drying of swamps, for example, eliminated mosquito breeding grounds and probably reduced the incidence of such mos-
quito-borne diseases as malaria and dengue fever. Likewise, the thorough
cleaning and whitewashing of medical buildings and vessels almost certainly contributed to the elimination of other disease-carrying vectors, such
as ticks, cockroaches, and mice. Alongside these measures, others of a more
superstitious character and unproven efficacy continued to be applied.
Regulating human behavior, for instance, was also a convenient way to consolidate control over new settlements along the African coast, and a resourceful tactic to govern vessels all throughout the Atlantic.

All in all, frustrations associated with the lack of success of many of
these measures, even those that almost certainly helped to ease the impact
of some diseases, were prevalent. Slave trading factories, anti–slave trade
reception centers, and in more general terms Western settlements along the
African coast—as well as many of those on the other side of the ocean—
were all subjected to morbid environments where human lives, including
those of the Africans, were hard to protect. At sea, the situation was often

the same, or perhaps even more desperate as numerous witnesses' accounts suggest.[128] Prophylactic and preventive measures may have ultimately saved lives, but it is beyond any doubt that they also served more complex agendas and interests. In more than one way they constituted both medical attempts to stop diseases from arriving and spreading and a backdoor for free trade and emerging colonial interests.

The Blood of Thousands

Slave Traders and the Fight against
Disease in the Age of Abolition

> ... before you left I begged you in God's name not to take the
> crazy decision of going to Africa.
> —Ysabel Klem to her son Ysidro Powell.
> Cárdenas, August 14, 1830

ON MAY 5, 1825, the crew of the French brig *Le Jeune Louis* gathered together shortly after their surgeon, Denis Béjaud, died of dysentery, the same disease that had killed the ship owners' representative on board, Jean-Baptiste Ménard, less than two weeks before. Probably sitting around a table in the captain's cabin, they set out to write and sign a short declaration in which they explained the despairing situation they found themselves in. As they sailed in the vicinity of Ascension Island heading for Cuba with a human cargo in their hold, they lamented the ravages that dysentery and ophthalmia had caused both to themselves and to the slaves. Affected by these two diseases—and probably also by others they did not mention—they attempted a head count of the remaining Africans, noting that out of the 344 they had embarked near Cape Formosa in the Bight of Biafra, 304 remained alive, but were all suffering from one or more diseases. At sea, far from their desired destination, and being "unable of caring for the cargo, and hardly able to manoeuver the vessel" due to the blindness caused by the ophthalmia, they probably thought that all was lost, as each of them signed his name on the small sheet of paper.[1]

By mid-June, however, 229 Africans and a handful of sailors, including the captain François Demouy, had made it alive to Havana, where the French consul, Jacques Marie Angelucci, and the cosignatories of the vessel took care of restoring their health and of justifying the voyage before the Spanish and French authorities, after producing many documents, which included the death certificates of a number of Africans. Before too long they also expedited the loading of the vessel, sending it back to Europe less than two months later with a cargo of sugar boxes belonging to Cuban planter and prominent slave trader Gabriel Lombillo.[2]

Perhaps better than any other, the case of *Le Jeune Louis* encapsulates the dangers associated with slave-trading expeditions to the coast of Africa during the illegal period that followed the signing of bilateral treaties between Britain and a number of slave-trading nations and states. Not only were the crew and the slaves exposed to fatal, debilitating, and incapacitating diseases, but within days of departing from the African coast they were left without the man responsible for the hundreds of slaves they had on board, and more significant, without their only health practitioner. In addition to all these tribulations, *Le Jeune Louis* had been previously stopped and searched at least twice by anti–slave trade patrols since departing from Bordeaux, and had been forced to remain in the Bight of Biafra for approximately four months, sailing back and forth to the island of Principe, until a full human cargo was finally procured.[3]

Slave ships like *Le Jeune Louis* turned into shared spaces where disease struck the overwhelming majority of those who were on board during the Middle Passage. That dysentery, ophthalmia, and fever attacked and claimed the lives of French slavers and enslaved African alike reveals the precariousness of human life and the limitations of medical treatment to combat these diseases. In particular, for the crew of *Le Jeune Louis,* spending four months in the Bight of Biafra seems to have become a death sentence for many: a long exposure to slave-trading contact zones, where diseases—tropical and otherwise—were exchanged on a regular basis took a large human toll, both among them and among the Africans they crammed in the bowels of the vessel.

Just as slave ships were shared spaces, slave factories and towns where interactions took place between African rulers, slave-trading factors, and slave-ship captains and crews became notoriously unhealthy spots where, along with the horrors of slavery and a variety of forms of human violence, potentially fatal diseases were always present. Whereas a number of surviving letters written by slave dealers during this period suggest that some of them went to great lengths to protect their human cargoes, others were much less interested in the conditions in which Africans were treated, traded, and transported across the ocean. The historical evidence available to historians indicates that the changes that took place in the slave trade after 1807 and particularly after 1820 led to even more human suffering, as slave dealers changed their modus operandi by taking concealing measures that had a direct effect on the treatment and health of the men, women, and children they assembled along the African coast to be sold into the transatlantic slave trade. In short, by engaging with the documentation left behind by slave dealers during this period, I reveal in this chapter that slave dealers both at sea and on land were just as likely to fall ill and die as the men, women, and children they were trafficking. I also scrutinize and discuss the ways in which slave traders fought back against debilitating and deadly diseases throughout the Atlantic world, revealing how, in spite of inhabiting an illegal realm, they often used state-of-the-art remedies and therapies that did not differ much from strategies used by those attempting to bring their slave-trading endeavors to an end.

Slave-Trading Expeditions and Lethal Diseases

From the minute slave vessels left from any of the American or European ports where they had been fitted for their ultimate purpose of trading slaves in Africa, apprehension about what was to come descended on all those involved. News about deceased slave-ship captains and sailors was common on both sides of the Atlantic. From Havana to Benguela, and from Barcelona to Rio de Janeiro, all those involved in the slave trade gossiped and lamented the loss of fellow slave dealers. As one slave-trade health practitioner ironically put it in a letter sent in 1830 after mentioning the deaths of two slave ship masters, Torrent and Vergallo, who had died after leaving for Havana from Gallinas and Bonny, respectively, "This is the common luck [that awaits us] in these, always very blessed lands."[4]

Slave-trading expeditions in the post-1820 Atlantic were tense and dangerous affairs. Along with the always-present risks of being seized by an anti–slave trade patrol cruiser, of being attacked and plundered by a pirate, or of sinking in an ocean storm, diseases constituted a further peril. Up and down the Atlantic and beyond, those who chose or were compelled to enter this inhuman business were continuously at the mercy of both diseases and their remedies, which were precarious and often just as deadly.

Most traders were well aware of the risks they were taking, as the reputation of the torrid zones, especially along the coast of Africa, was known in virtually every corner of an increasingly globalized Atlantic world. These fears were behind discussions, public and private, regarding the slave trade, at a time when the business had been outlawed by practically every Atlantic state on both sides of the ocean. An illustrative case of this kind was narrated by R. B. Estrada, a Cuban slave trader who visited Rio Pongo in the mid-1830s and who left a vexing narrative of his voyage to this infamous slave-trading haunt, and of the death of one of his shipmates.[5] Estrada's story concerned the fate of one Alonso Forest, the son of a French coffee plantation owner near Havana, who had been hired by the notorious slave dealer Paul Faber in Havana to travel to Bangalang to work as a bookkeeper in his factory. According to Estrada, before leaving for the coast of Africa, Forest's relatives attempted to dissuade him from taking such a hazardous employment, "such was the hatred and terror that the coast of Africa and its dreaded consequences had upon them."[6] Against their objections and premonitions, he insisted that, providing he did not die, the salary Faber was offering—two thousand pesos and twelve slaves per year—would allow him to return home a rich man within two or three years. As it happened, Forest lasted exactly thirteen days. Estrada, who also suffered from fevers and dysentery at the same time, recalled that Forest had died in his arms, a victim of the climate of Rio Pongo.[7]

In a similar case, Ysabel Klem, the mother of another nineteenth-century slave trader, Ysidro Powell, questioned in various letters sent to her son his reasons for abandoning her in order to pursue the life of a slaver. Powell had left for Rio Pongo in early 1829 to work alongside Edward Jousiffe, another leading slave dealer at that spot, and by 1830 news about the poor state of his

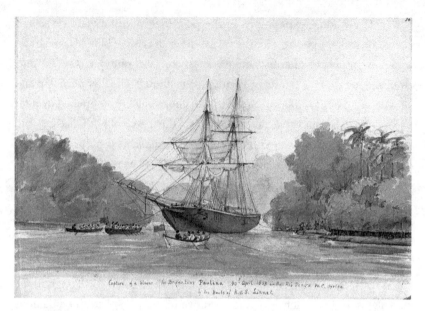

Fig. 7. Capture of slaver *Paulina* in Rio Pongo. NMM: Album. Art/10. MS65/134.

health had traversed the Atlantic to his mother, who had stayed behind in Cárdenas taking care of the family's businesses. On August 30, 1830, Klem reproached her son's silence and begged him to write her a letter, after having referred to his voyage to Africa as "crazy" only a few days before.[8]

While relatives lived in fear, expecting devastating news any time, those who embarked on slave ships, or who settled along the coast of Africa, had to confront diseases as part of their daily lives. Plenty of letters and testimonies from slave dealers of this period have survived until today, giving us an insight into the ways in which they thought of diseases and accepted them as an inescapable menace and the ways in which they fought against them, including the medicines and treatments they used before, during, and after loading their ships with their human cargo.

Before departing for Africa, slave captains throughout the period were always given specific sets of instructions pertaining the particulars of their voyages. These instructions could cover a wide variety of matters, including the routes they were expected to follow on their voyage to Africa and upon their return, the best places for dealing in human beings in Africa

and for landing them in the Americas, the names of agents placed in different Atlantic spots in cases of emergency landings, the flag combinations
they were expected to follow, and the manner in which they were expected
to treat their crew and the Africans once these had been brought on board.

Slave Ships

Slave ships were archetypical contact zones. On them, African slaves and
their captors lived in a common, reduced space for weeks or months at a
time, sharing air and fluids. As a result, a diverse variety of viruses and bac-
teria were also exchanged. By the time the slave trade was declared illegal in
the early nineteenth century, health practitioners throughout the Atlantic
knew this all too well. They were aware of the dangers associated with sharing such spaces at sea, far from any other medical facilities, and they often
discussed them in their work.

    The reality was that the slave ship's environment was just as lethal as
the geographical ecosystems where the diseases carried on board had originated. This was especially the case after the slave trade was banned by most
of the Atlantic states from the mid-1810s onward. The resulting modifications in the shipping and accommodation of Africans on slave vessels as a
result of the work of anti–slave trade patrols led to hurried processes of loading the ships, often overlooking such thorough health inspections of enslaved men, women, and children as had taken place in the previous decades.
These changes were widely discussed at the time by anti–slave trade cruisers, by diplomatic officers, and even by slave dealers across the Atlantic.

    Although slave vessels' sizes, speed, and conditions on board changed
at times dramatically over the years, the existing historical evidence points
to an overall worsening of the conditions during the Middle Passage after
the slave trade became illegal. Regardless of their respective sizes, overcrowding became a main feature of the slave trade during this period.
Practically every one of the documented voyages for these years reveals
ghastly conditions on board. Reduced and dirty spaces for human habita-
tion, lacking clean air; spoiled water and food; punishment, tortures,
and rapes; ever longer journeys; slave revolts; encounters with privateers,

pirates, and anti-slave trade patrols; and particularly the ravages of disease—all combined to create some of the most desperate conditions ever experienced by human beings in the modern world.

Slave dealers were not impervious to some of these episodes and maladies, either. The instructions they were almost always given at the start of their transatlantic voyages suggest that investors and owners of slave-trading expeditions were keen to avoid risks, particularly those concerning the possible spread of harmful diseases among their human cargo. This, for example, was the reasoning behind the contract signed in Santiago de Cuba by slave-ship captain Mariano Carbó in November 1819. Not only did he—and his sailors—agree to forfeit every penny of their salary should the ship wreck, but they also agreed to "take care of the *negrada* [human cargo] with the greatest attentiveness and cleanliness, without complaining about any foulness, and regardless of the diseases they [the Africans] could be suffering from."[9]

The instructions given to Carbó were similar to those received by other contemporary slave-ship captains. Just a year before they were issued, well-known slave trader and owner Gabriel Lombillo reminded the captain of the ship *Campeador,* Ramón Ozquiano, that "cleaning and scouring are very necessary at all times . . . because if you do not have this precaution, they could have a pest that would affect the expedition."[10] Lombillo also suggested that Ozquiano's crew should bathe the slaves every morning in order to "free them from diseases," and treat them with all the possible care, feeding them well so that they would not lose too much weight in the Middle Passage, a circumstance that should be avoided at all costs, because should they arrive too thin, it would "make selling them difficult."[11]

In a similar vein in 1839 the captain of the Brazilian vessel *Especulador,* Francisco Jozé de Abranxes, was prompted to carry out a slave-trading voyage to Anha, in Mozambique, making sure that the slaves he transported would arrive in the best possible conditions, as the ship owner, Jozé Joaquim Teixeira, confessed to be tired of suffering setbacks in his slave-trading expeditions.[12] Almost at the same time, in Havana, Pedro Martínez recommended slave-ship captain Andrés Jiménez—later on main slave dealer at the Gallinas River—"to treat the *bultos* [slaves] as well as he could," since his job would be judged according to the conditions in which they would arrive.[13] Jiménez was also strongly encouraged to use his experience in order to avoid any possible slave revolts during the Middle Passage.[14]

In spite of the occasional efforts to take care of human beings who were unavoidably crammed within small, filthy, hot spaces, diseases were a main feature of the Middle Passage. In order to fight health practitioners often shipped on slave vessels to look after both the human cargo and the crew. In some cases, these practitioners were Westerners who had received medical education in Europe or the Americas. On the *Voladora*, in 1829, the surgeon was one "Doctor Juan Hidalgo," a native of Rota, near Cádiz, who was said to be "unmarried and a professor of medicine and surgery."[15] Likewise, when in 1854 the ship *La Luisa* was captured off the mouth of the Manatí River near Trinidad in southern Cuba, the vessel's surgeon, Joaquim Cordeiro Feijóo, was said to be a member of the Society of Medical Sciences in Lisbon and an experienced surgeon who had been attached to the Portuguese troops in Luanda in previous years.[16]

In most cases, however, health practitioners seemed to have come from more humble backgrounds, and some ship officers, boatswains, or cooks doubled as surgeons on board of slave vessels.[17] African-born and Creole practitioners, called *sangradores,* were the norm for many expeditions during the period. For example, in 1821, Alexander Cunningham and Henry Hayne, British Mixed Commission court judges in Rio de Janeiro, had the opportunity to interrogate a man named José Joaquim de Moraes, who was described as a free black or *preto forro* "of Gêge nation," who confessed to be a "schooner's sangrador," a profession for which he was officially registered at Rio de Janeiro.[18] Manoel Francisco Silva, also an African-born free man of Gêge nation, worked as a sangrador on board the brig *Bom Caminho* two years later, while Estanislao Ysidro, a Creole born in Brazil, was recorded as the sangrador of the schooner *Bela Eliza*, in 1824.[19] Sangradores were usually African-born or African-descended health practitioners who had applied and attained official licenses from the Brazilian authorities to exercise their bloodletting knowledge on land and at sea.[20] According to Tânia Salgado Pimenta, sangradores were at times "the only therapeutic recourse for those who were sick" on board ships, thus becoming essential for the success of Portuguese and Brazilian slave-trade expeditions to Africa after 1820.[21]

Until recently we knew very little about the social and cultural extraction of the array of men who worked as health practitioners on board slave-
trade vessels after 1820.[22] Based on the names of the few we have been able
to identify, it seems that the majority of them were born in Europe or the
Americas. Some of them were described as "doctors" by those who recalled
meeting them or who described their activities. The cases of Juan Hidalgo,
Joaquím Cordeiro Feijóo, and Denis Béjaud were not unique, and as a matter of fact, some of them not only joined slave-trade expeditions but also
became slave dealers. Among those European- or American-educated physicians who entered the slave trade was Hanoverian doctor Daniel Botefeur,
who began his slave-trading career during the first years of the nineteenth
century. Botefeur, whose case has been well studied, engaged in human trafficking in the first few decades of the nineteenth century in the Upper
Guinea coast, along with notorious slave-trading factors like John Ormond
Jr. and Stiles Edward Lightbourn.[23]

Another health practitioner turned into slave-trade surgeon and eventually slave dealer during the period was French medical doctor Alphonse
Meynier. Meynier's career as a slave dealer spanned more than two decades,
and according to British captain Henry James Matson, who met him per-
sonally in the late 1840s, had begun soon after he was appointed a surgeon
for the British Navy in the late 1820s. Apparently dejected over the amount
of work he was being asked to do, and the poor financial rewards he received for it, Meynier decided to change careers. After becoming a slave
trader, he eventually settled near Ponta de Lenha at the Congo River, acting
as an agent for Havana-based fellow French slave trader Pedro Forçade.[24]

The daily work of sangradores, surgeons, and other health practitioners was a harrowing one, fraught with deadly hazards and meager rewards.
Slave-trading crews and the slaves they embarked were often the victims of
endemic and epidemic diseases difficult to diagnose and treat, even when
medical supplies were available. A number of narratives and documents, including correspondence, left by slave traders illustrate the environment to
which health practitioners and their patients were exposed. References were
common to sick and dead captains and crew members—including health
practitioners. In one such case, the captain of the American vessel *Senator*,

John Kelly, was reported to have died upon his arrival in Loango in 1847, almost certainly the victim of a severe case of yellow fever, which was ravaging the place at the time of the ship's arrival. According to William Laurenson and William Henry Christie, two of the *Senator*'s sailors, both slaves and crew were "very sick with the fever" on their passage to Brazil afterward. As a result, more than two hundred Africans died and all but three sailors spent the Middle Passage suffering and convalescing from the fevers.[25]

In another case, Antonio Puga, the captain of the Spanish schooner *Josefina,* was attacked by the "African fever" shortly after arriving in Gallinas in 1838, leading a slave-trading expedition organized by José Quevedo in Havana. After reaching his destination and establishing contact with Pablo Álvarez Simidel, one of the main agents of Cuban houses in the region, Puga found himself confined to what would be his deathbed. In a farewell letter to a friend in Havana, he bequeathed a watch and a chain so that the friend would have something to remember him by, after acknowledging that his days were "about to be ended in the tomb."[26]

African slaves fared much worse. The stories about lack of medical attention, bad treatment, and unspeakable abuses of different kinds that are discussed in the pages of this book testify to the horrors of the Middle Passage in the illegal period. Some slave traders described at length their experiences in dealing with the effects of disease among the slaves they carried across the ocean. The experiences of the *Senator*'s sailors provide us with a perfect example. When examined upon their return to Brazil in 1847, most of them felt compelled to refer to the sufferings of the Africans they had carried to Brazil. One of them, Joseph Alvares Cunha, described the Africans as having been brought on board and "stowed away like cargo in the hold." Cunha also revealed some details about their conditions of existence during the Middle Passage. For example, he pointed out that they "were allowed to come on deck for air about twice a week," and blamed their high mortality—246 out of 914 died in the Middle Passage—to the "scarcity of water."[27] Cunha's statement about the lack of water supplies was confirmed by William Laurenson, who added that on the first night at sea alone, 74 slaves had died, mostly due to "the want of water."[28] Laurenson added that these deaths of "men, women and children" were also a consequence of "the deck and hold being as full as they could be."[29]

The private letters written by some of the slave-ship captains of the period to their employers and partners also shed light on the morbidity and mortality that often affected those men, women, and children they carried against their will across the ocean. The captain of the Brazilian schooner-brig *Aracaty*, Joaquim Antônio Lima, in a letter sent to his partner Joaquim Pereira de Mendonça in early 1842, described in detail the loss of several hundred slaves on his previous slaving expedition to Africa, and reported losing a number of slaves on his present voyage before being detained by a British man-of-war after departing for Rio de Janeiro.[30] In a similar incident, the crew of the *Vigilante*, a Spanish slave vessel that had been attempting to get a human cargo near Cape Lopez in 1838, sailed at once for Santiago de Cuba after the captain concluded that there was no point in remaining any longer off the coast of Africa, as the slaves they had bought were dying faster than they were able to replace them.[31]

The cases of other equally full and lethal slave ships filled the reports of Mixed Commission and Vice-Admiralty courts, often leading to renewed calls for the abolition of the slave trade. Rarely, however, did the Africans have the opportunity to describe their own traumatic experiences in the Middle Passage. One of the few exceptions was the case of Antonio and Dominga, two young Africans—about eleven or twelve years old—who had been sold and embarked at the port of Boma on the Congo River, sometime in late 1857 or early 1858. Antonio and Dominga, whose real names were Bata and Manyeré Curo, recounted their difficult time before Spanish colonial officers in Havana weeks after their arrival. They testified that during the Middle Passage they were given only one cracker per day, and "that they were all very hungry, that they would ask for something to eat, and they would get nothing."[32] They also recounted that as many as fifty of their companions had died of disease and hunger, and that their bodies had all been invariably "thrown to the sea."[33]

The testimonies of the Africans taken from river Gallinas in 1838 on board the schooner *Arrogante* were even more striking, as some of them accused the ship's sailors of murdering one of the Africans, and of subsequently cooking his flesh and serving it with rice to the rest of the slaves.[34] They also accused the sailors of reserving the murdered man's heart and liver for their own consumption, in what it was one of the few documented cases of likely cannibalism in the history of the transatlantic slave trade. Nor did the accusations leveled against the *Arrogante*'s crew stop there, as the sailors were also accused of torturing and murdering many more, of raping several women, and of denying medical attention to those who fell ill during the Middle Passage.[35]

Conditions on slave factories along the coast of Africa, and on occasion on the landing spots in the Americas, were often just as challenging for both slave dealers and for the men, women, and children they enslaved and trafficked. The temporary slave prisons known as barracoons had a particular reputation for being deadly holding areas where Africans could spend months at a time, and where many among them met their final fate.

Factories, Urban Centers, and Barracoons

In 1848 Lieutenant Frederick Barnard published an account of his first three years on board an anti-slave trade patrol vessel in Africa.[36] In 1842 Barnard had been assigned to serve under the orders of Captain Christopher Wyvill on HMS *Cleopatra*, one of the ships of the Cape of Good Hope squadron, a position he would continue to hold until he was reassigned in 1845.[37]

Barnard's account of his time cruising off the East African coast in search of slavers features some of the most gripping passages ever written about the human suffering that slave traders caused, both at sea and on land. In one of his earlier recollections, Barnard described going on land to visit the town of Quelimane in February 1843 and finding that "Every thing appeared to denote the unavoidable existence of fever and disease."[38] From that moment on, a sequence of accidents, instances of bad treatment, and references to fatal diseases appeared in his narrative, highlighting the dreadful conditions existing on the barracoons and in small slave-trading towns along this coast, where slaves could usually be seen looking like "mere skeletons, with death depicted in their countenances."[39] Only three or four days after he had returned to the *Cleopatra* from visiting Quelimane, he noted that "300 slaves had been burnt alive in a baracoon some distance to the northward, where they had been sent ready for embarkation."[40] He then reflected on the cruel behavior exhibited by the slave dealers and on their stratagems to circumvent British efforts to stop them from trading in human beings. Finally, Barnard recounted in horror having witnessed the loading, sailing, and swift return of a black schooner belonging to a "Senhor Isidoro." Barnard recalled that more than four hundred Africans had been crammed on board the said ship up the river at Macuze, and that soon after leaving the coast, the master had been forced to order her return after losing "one-half of her human cargo" from disease, landing again "the wretched remnant half death."[41]

Distressing as they were, Barnard's recollections about daily occurrences in slave-trading spots along the African coast were far from unique. Many other narratives point to these sites as dangerous places, where disease was a permanent feature, and where other hazards, including armed attacks—both from land and from the sea—slave uprisings, kidnappings, and escapes were also frequent. Long periods spent in barracoons or factories after demanding walks from the interior regions, enforced daily labor while waiting to be embarked, and the unreliability of medical attention and facilities combined to create some of the most perilous sites throughout the Atlantic world at the time.[42]

Although there were clear differences between slave-trading urban settlements such as Ouidah, Cabinda, or Benguela and more rustic factories concealed within less-populated coastal areas, like those found throughout the period at rivers Pongo, Gallinas, and Congo, they all, invariably, turned into model slave-trade contact zones. The same could be said about slave-trade landing sites on the American side of the Atlantic, where once again, those who had arrived on slave ships—often suffering from debilitating and lethal diseases—came into close contact with local dealers and residents.

Unlike infirmaries and other medical facilities, which were often lacking, barracoons were ever-present in slave-trade contact zones. References to these barracoons are plentiful. Those built at the rivers of Guinea were frequently described by visitors and by anti–slave trade patrol officers, who on occasion attacked and destroyed them. At Ouidah there were at least six large barracoons in the mid-1840s, which were reportedly located in the vi-

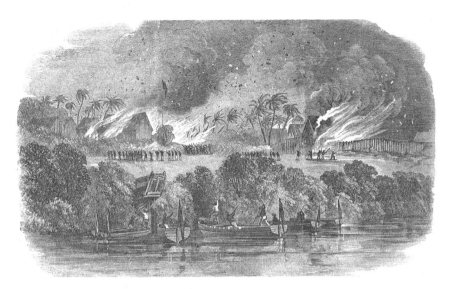

Fig. 8. Destruction of barracoons in Mozambique. *Illustrated London News,* January 18, 1851.

cinity of the residence of Francisco Félix de Souza, the main slave trader there.[43] At other slave trade sites like the Congo River, Cabinda, Loango, Ambriz, Ambrizette, and Benguela, slave barracoons were a permanent feature of the landscape at least from the late eighteenth century, being the subject of several reports and stories related to the slave trade in these territories.[44]

Slave barracoons along the coasts of West, West Central, and East Africa were at once sites of extreme oppression and repositories of disease. The conditions of existence in them were so obviously desperate that even those who were highly critical of the situation on board slave vessels were at times keen to point out that living standards at these barracoons were just as bad as or even worse than those they had observed on slave ships. In 1850, British diplomat William Gore Ouseley called barracoons "pestilent" and condemned the "destructive marches over immense tracts of desert" that later resulted in "starvation and crowding" on these sites.[45]

In many of them, slaves were kept enclosed within fenced pens, where movement was limited and where the heat of the tropical sun exacerbated their exhaustion and health afflictions. Even when slaves were allowed out, forced labor often ensued.[46] This was the case in the Rio Pongo barracoons belonging to such slave traders as John Ormond Jr., Stiles Edward Lightbourn, Tom Curtis, and Paul Faber. According to a number of Africans who were interviewed by the British authorities in Freetown in 1822, temporary enforced labor while waiting for embarkation was a common occurrence in most of the barracoons there.[47] Sulimana, a Foulah from Yimboo, who was seized on board the Spanish schooner *Rosalia* in 1822, declared that from the time of his arrival at Bangalang, he had been "employed in filling water casks to put on board the vessel," and that whenever he was not forced to work, he was in chains, "long chains, twenty slaves upon one chain and fifteen upon the other."[48] Sulimana's testimony was backed by that of Jumo, from Jalonka, who also mentioned the chains they were all put in, and referred to the hard labor they were subjected to, filling out water casks for the slave vessels.[49]

As a matter of fact, lines of chained African slaves waiting to be embarked along African beaches were described by slave traders almost as frequently as they were by anti–slave trade patrol officers. German slave-trade investor C. H. Von Zütphen told of one such group of chained men, women, and children he had seen while expecting to ship a human cargo in the Bight of Benin in the early 1830s. They were, he wrote, "taken by the beach towards the barracoons in groups of 30, lined up and chained by their necks."[50] Similarly, in 1844, some of the sailors belonging to the American brig *Sea Eagle* reported seeing "droves of negroes" who came "down to the shore" at Cabinda in similar circumstances to those described by Von Zütphen years before.[51] James Fawkner, who visited West Africa in 1825 as the captain of the merchant vessel *Nymph,* also left a dreary account of the moment he came across a group of slaves belonging to the King of Popo who had just been released from a barracoon:

> The slaves when they made their appearance exhibited a long line of melancholy faces and emaciated frames, wasted by disease and close confinement, and by having suffered dreadfully from scantiness of food, and the impure air of the prison house. They were 231 in number, men, women, and children; in a com-

plete state of nudity and heavily manacled. Several of them were lamed by the weight of their irons, and their skin sadly excoriated from the same cause.[52]

Overcrowding in particular became a major problem for the health of the slaves, and also of the slave dealers, as the efforts of anti–slave trade patrols became more systematic and effective. The obligatory waiting time in congested barracoons, which could last for months, created an environment conducive to the spread of numerous infectious diseases. British personnel engaged in attacking and destroying barracoons along the coast of Africa were well aware of the drawbacks resulting from their aggressive policies. In a letter sent to London in 1844, Mixed Commission court officers at Freetown Michael Melville and James Hook expressed their concern about the success that British Navy cruisers had had in dissuading slave ships from carrying on their usual trade in the region. An unwanted consequence of this success, they noted, was that an accumulation of slaves was "reported to have occurred in several barracoons, occasioning much disease and mortality, from the crowded state of these places and a scarcity of food."[53] This assessment was confirmed both by French anti–slave trade squadron officers and by the slave traders themselves. In a letter sent in 1845, French Commander Auguste Baudin confirmed the opinion of Melville and Hook when he mentioned that Andrés Jiménez's barracoons in Gallinas were all "full of blacks who were only waiting for a chance to be embarked."[54] In the same vein, just a few years earlier, in 1838, Melville and Hook's predecessors, H. W. Macaulay and R. Doherty, portrayed a remarkably similar scenario when they described the slave barracoons at river Gallinas as overloaded spaces. In their opinion the reason behind this desperate situation was the efficiency of the navy in capturing slavers, which had forced the local slave dealers to limit their captives "almost to a starvation allowance of food."[55] They also remarked that this circumstance, combined with "their close confinement, and their being heavily ironed had produced extensive mortality among them."[56] Theodore Canot, who was one of those slave dealers to be affected by these aggressive policies, confirmed the statement of the Mixed Commission officers when he wrote years later about the famine and death that such a blockade had created in his barracoons at River Sestos in the early 1840s.[57]

By the final years of the transatlantic slave trade the situation was even more desperate for the Africans who had been sent to the barracoons on the coast. In December 1864, Commodore Arthur Eardley Wilmot pointed out in a letter sent to the Admiralty officers in London that hundreds of slaves had been waiting to be shipped in some of "the principal depôts on the coast," and that they were being "constantly marched from place to place . . . but without success."[58] The combination of repeated marches and of long delays at barracoons had, in his opinion, "led to great mortality amongst them, from privations and disease of every kind."[59] Anti–slave trade patrol attacks also led on occasion to rushed retreats into the interior, which almost certainly resulted in further human suffering and deaths. Some of the slaves seized on board of the *Rosalia* in 1822 mentioned that upon the arrival of the British at Bangalang, they had been concealed in haste by Ormond, who sent half of them to the house of a man named Bougali, where they remained hidden until further notice.[60] In a similar instance, French Commander Auguste Baudin reported finding the slave barracoons at Cape Mount empty, as the slave dealers in that place had been warned of his arrival and had arranged for a speedy escape into the interior with all of the slaves.[61]

Forced labor, bad treatment, overcrowding, and famine were not, however, the only factors affecting morbidity and mortality levels in these factories along the coast. In slave factories like those situated in some of the rivers of Upper Guinea, medical facilities were poor or practically nonexistent, and medical attention was rudimentary. Even in more developed urban centers like those of Ouidah, Onim, Cabinda, or Benguela, the pestilent conditions alluded to by Ouseley had a direct effect on slave dealers and on the crews of the slave ships they traded with. The testimony of R. B. Estrada, who decided to tell his story in Havana after returning from a slave-trading voyage to Rio Pongo, sheds light on the conditions faced by all those living in factories along the coast of Africa. In addition to the premature death of his fellow traveler and friend Alonso Forest, Estrada recalled several episodes that revealed how disease hindered the lives of those who trafficked in human beings in the factories built along this river.

One of them referred to the *Narcisa,* a Spanish slave vessel that had arrived in Rio Pongo shortly before Estrada's own ship, the *Gaceta.* To Estrada's surprise, at the time of his arrival the *Narcisa* was fully under the control of four of Paul Faber's men, who had been tasked with taking care of it while the master, the notorious slave-ship captain Santiago Comas, the first mate, and a few surviving sailors recovered from the fevers that had already killed most of the *Narcisa*'s crew. Estrada was hardly exaggerating when he noted down that any foreigner landing on the place would last four days at most before being attacked by the fevers.[62] Estrada himself, and most of the crew of the *Gaceta,* fell victims of the fevers a few days later, just as they sailed away, attempting to reach San Vicente, in the Cape Verde islands, where they had planned to wait a few days while their human cargo was readied for embarkation. Surviving the fevers, however, was only a partial victory, as they were soon followed by bouts of dysentery, which only subsided after the vessel took its enslaved cargo and sailed back to Cuba.[63]

Factories and other urban settlements involved in the transatlantic slave trade became, in fact, the final resting places for many of the slave dealers from Europe and the Americas who decided to travel to the African coast and to conduct their business from there. Among those who found their death there was Juan José Zangroniz Jr., one of the leading slave traders of the period, whose reputation as a main dealer at Ouidah was comparable to that of Francisco Félix de Souza.[64] Zangroniz, who had moved to Ouidah at some point between 1831 and 1833 to become the African-based agent of his family firm Zangroniz Brothers & Co., died in 1843 in his mid-thirties, probably as a result of an attack of fever.[65] In previous years he, like virtually every other Westerner settled along the coast, had found himself frequently ill and in a debilitated condition. In a letter sent in 1836 to Miguel Palau, the master of one of the slave ships sent to Ouidah by his relatives in Havana, he confessed not to be aware of "what had been going on outside," as he had been too ill to leave his quarters.[66]

In a similar case, Antonio Jordi, a Catalonian factor who became the main slave dealer at Little Bassam in the late 1820s and early 1830s, lamented in his letters to Antonio González Carbajal, his partner at Grand Bassam, that the health of the other white dealers who worked alongside him at the place was very poor. In his own words, his French competitor at Little Bassam—whose name was never mentioned—was repeatedly "sick" to the point that Jordi confessed to being sorry for him.[67] At some point Jordi also mentioned in his letters that both Ramón—who was probably his main partner—and "the Portuguese man" who also worked for him were of no use, as they were both continuously ill.[68]

On the American side of the ocean conditions were marginally better, free of some of the most debilitating and deadly diseases endemic to the African coast. Even so, barracoons and other equally oppressive detention areas were also permanent features along the coasts of the main importers of slaves in the period, Brazil and Cuba. Even the barracoons of the city of Havana—a mixed sort of pseudolegal and illegal depots—where recently landed Africans arguably received a more sophisticated treatment, mostly in order to fatten them to improve their salability, reflected this dreadful reality. British diplomat and abolitionist David Turnbull, who visited some of them in the late 1830s, mentioned that it was "the policy of the importer to restore as soon as possible, among the survivors the strength that has been wasted and the health that had been lost during the horrors of the middle passage," in order to fetch higher prices once they were put for sale.[69] Throughout the period the barracoons were considered as unhealthy sites, and Africans who arrived in the city and its surroundings particularly sick were usually taken to the lazaretto that had been established in the Vedado neighborhood, outside of the city limits.[70]

Across the island, even within major urban centers like Havana, Matanzas, and Santiago de Cuba, other more precarious barracoons were prepared to receive human cargoes from Africa, known in Cuba as *alijos*. Many sites were located within the boundaries of sugar plantations near the coast. Some of the most important sugar planters of the period, including Bernabé Martínez de Pinillos, Juan Miró Pié, and Salvador Martiartu, were among those at whose plantations slave-ship captains were often instructed to deliver the Africans they had transported across the Atlantic. In 1854, for example, the authorities of Güines, a village located south of Havana, found a number of dying Africans resting on a beach alongside some of the slave dealers who had brought them to Cuba. When the authorities examined the area, they encountered three precarious structures to which the Africans were supposed to have been taken. Nearby, they also noticed soil that had been recently dug, almost certainly indicating that some of them had been buried there.[71]

Some of the British diplomats based in the Cuban capital did, on occasion, pay incognito visits to the barracoons of the city, in order to report on their whereabouts and the living conditions they offered those who were imprisoned in them.[72] In the midst of the cholera epidemic that struck western Cuba in 1833, slave ships and the slaves they had brought from Africa were, once again, blamed for the origin and spread of a new terrifying disease. The paper trail resulting from two events that transpired during that summer revealed to a certain extent how barracoons built on the countryside to receive newly arrived slaves played an essential role for the successful completion of slave-trading expeditions.

The first of these events, an African armed insurgency, took place on August 13 in the district of Banes, west of Havana. A combination of newly arrived Lucumí (in their majority Yoruba) Africans who had been placed on the slave barracoons of the coffee estate Salvador, belonging to a notorious Basque slave trader and planter, joined forces with some other Lucumís who had been living on the plantation for some time.[73] Together they created a daunting military unit, which invaded and ransacked several plantations in the region until they were finally defeated by a combined force of the regular army and local militias. In the aftermath, it became apparent that these former Lucumí soldiers had been reunited only because the plantation owner, Francisco Santiago Aguirre, had used some of the barracoons that would normally have been reserved for plantation slaves to house hundreds of recently arrived Africans who were to have been sold to other planters of the region, a sale from which he expected a substantial profit.[74]

The second event took place south of Havana, in the town of Bejucal, only a few days later. This time, another group of recently arrived slaves was "deposited in the Barracon of a well-known Catalan slave dealer under powerful private protection."[75] Although this time there was no uprising, the local residents, fearful of the possibility of sharing space with a group of Africans who they believed were carriers of cholera, wrote letters of complaint to

Captain General Ricafort and demanded that the local authorities remove the Africans from their neighborhood.

Although these barracoons often doubled as slave markets, where prospective owners could visit and choose those men, women, and children they desired to buy, on occasion sales were made right after landings had taken place, doubtless in order to avoid likely losses that could result from postlanding mortality among the new arrivals. British traveler Henry Tudor commented on this when he visited Matanzas in the early 1830s. At the city docks he witnessed the public auction of a human cargo that had just arrived at the port from the African continent. Later he referred to the "stony-hearted speculators on human flesh" he had observed bidding for the Africans, including some who were lying on the ground and considered to be terminally ill.[76]

In addition to purpose-built barracoons, in many instances special houses in cities and the countryside were equipped to receive large numbers of slaves. In both cases, medical attention and medical facilities were limited, although for those Africans seized by British antislavery patrols, the hospitals and lazarettos of the city, and from the late 1830s onward HMS *Romney,* were put at their disposition. Just like the barracoons, some of these houses were also visited and described by British diplomats living in Havana. The Liberated African Department superintendent in Havana, Richard Robert Madden, reported one such case in 1836, when he wrote to his colleague Edward Schenley informing him about a cargo of Congo slaves who had been landed in the vicinity of the city and who had then been marched to a house in Oficios Street in the heart of the city, where they all had been subsequently purchased by the hatters firm of Manzaneda and Abusquete.[77] Less than a year later, both Schenley and Madden wrote to Captain General Miguel Tacón, reporting another sale of *bozal*—recently arrived Africans—slaves at a house in the Paseo del Prado, no. 61, which had taken place under the eyes of the Spanish authorities.[78]

Along the vast Brazilian coastline, from the northern Amazonian regions to the southernmost provinces, barracoons and other custom-made depositories were also used to receive large numbers of often-sick African slaves. A number of cases from this period reveal that houses of individuals who resided near the Atlantic coast were usually employed to receive groups of African slaves.[79] One of these places was the house of notorious slave dealer Vicente Paula e Silva in the neighborhood of Caes Dourado in Salvador. African slaves landed in various points of the coast in the vicinity of Salvador would be occasionally forced to endure long marches to slave traders' houses in the lower city. One such landing took place in 1833, when the Africans who had arrived in the brig-schooner *Atrevido* were disembarked at the creek of Itapagipe, and from there were taken to Paula e Silva's house, "into which they were admitted about 4 o'clock in the morning" of the following day.[80] As had been the case in Cuba, barracoons were also a regular feature, both in cities and in the countryside. In Rio de Janeiro, for example, recently arrived Africans were placed in barracoons known as *casas de engorda*—fattening houses—where they were fed and where their diseases were treated in the hope of helping them recover enough so that they could be sold at the highest possible prices.[81]

Medical attention and facilities in these landing spots were regularly administered poorly, and those African slaves and slave-ship crews who arrived sick had little recourse but to continue with treatments similar to those they had received during the Middle Passage. In some exceptional occasions, however, slave dealers set up more advanced medical buildings and routines in order to help the slaves and the crews recover from the long Atlantic crossings. This was the case of the brig *Paez*, taken to Cárdenas in 1857, with a number of African slaves who were considered to be very ill. As soon as the local authorities were made aware of the situation, they ordered that a reception center should be built in the outer rim of the harbor, in Cayo Diana, in order to avoid any possible contagion to the town's population. It was also determined that the reception center should have four barracoons, two large ones for the Africans, one to function as an infirmary, and a final one for the white crew of the brig.[82] Thanks to the testimonies of a number of American sailors who were interviewed in Rio de Janeiro in the mid-1840s, we know of at least one similar case. After denouncing the slave-trading businesses of Domingos Ruiz Souto, the American vice-consul in Vitoria, Espiritu Santo, sailors John Fairburn and James Gillespie pointed out that Souto had "at Victoria an Hospital for the treatment and cure of slaves arriving sick from the Coast of Africa."[83]

All in all, different locations and business models could have a direct or indirect impact on the overall conditions of the Africans and their captors and traders on both sides of the Atlantic.[84] Ultimately, however, health practitioners who were in charge of diagnosing and treating both slaves and slave traders were the protagonists of the fight against disease throughout the Atlantic world. Their work, whether done for good or for evil, was central to the functioning of the slave trade during the illegal period, as they attempted to treat diseases with their limited resources in the hope of obtaining bigger margins of profits for themselves and for their employers.

Fighting Disease: Remedies and Treatments

On August 28, 1828, the Spanish frigate *Veloz Pasagera* left from Havana bound for the port of Ouidah in West Africa in a slave-trading expedition. Before arriving at its final destination in June 1830, the ship touched on a number of African coastal towns in order to replenish its supplies of food and water. Coming into close proximity with African contact zones eventually reflected on the health on board. Not long after the vessel's arrival in Ouidah, the captain, José Antonio de la Vega, went on land and subsequently spent several months fighting for his life, treated by two Spanish health practitioners.

In the first of several letters sent from Ouidah by Luciano Belloch, one of these two practitioners, he confirmed to Alejandro Nocetti, the *Veloz Pasagera*'s first mate, who had been left in charge of the vessel, that the captain had spent the previous nine days in bed. In Belloch's opinion, de la Vega had been the victim of a sunstroke, which had mutated into a sequence of feverish attacks that were being treated with a combination of purgatives, emetics, and leeches.[85] Over the next few days, Belloch's reports of the captain's deteriorating health and of his attempts to arrest the advancement of de la Vega's maladies became more somber, as well as more explicative. On June 23, Belloch again administered an emetic remedy, which served to temporarily improve de la Vega's condition. This medication was followed later that day by the application of leeches to the stomach, and by a bath of water with malva leaves and vinegar. Seeing that nothing worked, Belloch gave the captain plenty of orange juice and decided, in conjunction with a colleague, to bleed him profusely from fourteen cuts he made to his neck and head with a lancet.[86]

In the following days the captain began to show some signs of improvement. By June 27 Belloch noticed that the captain was much better, but that he was now suffering from hemorrhoids, which were making him "rabid." In order to cure them, Belloch began using blistering plasters, more baths of water of malva leaves, and liniments—specifically, unguents of populeon and basilicon—all of which proved ineffective.[87] By the beginning of July, Belloch was running out of remedies to treat de la Vega's hemorrhoids. To the strategies he had mentioned previously he now added steam baths, various oily ointments, and baths of okra, and complained that the best two possible remedies he could think of, milk and leeches, were impossible to procure at the time, making his work much more difficult.[88]

A little less than a week later, the captain was back in bed and Belloch himself was now affected by a violent fever. Nicolás Calveras, who replaced Belloch while he was unable to perform his duties, wrote to Nocetti on July 7, reporting that the doctor had been suffering from "high temperature, cold [shivering] and vomits," while the captain's condition had become critical. Belloch himself managed to write a couple of lines that day, confirming the condition of the captain and letting Nocetti know that he was also very sick with "fever and vomiting bile."[89]

Over the next few weeks, Calveras continued to inform Nocetti about the poor health of both patients. At some point he complained about the situations he was confronting both on land and on board the *Veloz Pasagera*, referring to the ship as a "marine hospital" and to his own quarters in Ouidah as "another hospital."[90] Only at the beginning of August did Belloch begin to improve enough to recount the events of the previous weeks, reporting that he had been sick with fever for most of July, but that he was now finally getting better. The captain, on the other hand, was looking much weaker and feeble, a circumstance that made him think that "a very fatal outcome" was likely in his case.[91] In spite of such a gloomy prognosis, de la Vega made a full recovery and soon after was arrested by the British while trying to cross the Atlantic with a human cargo in the hold of his ship.[92]

The same ordeal to which José Antonio de la Vega and Luciano Belloch were subjected played out all across the illegal Atlantic until the end of
the transatlantic slave trade in the late 1860s. Medical treatments were regularly administered by health practitioners according to their knowledge of
medicine and the availability of medical supplies, which were not always
forthcoming, particularly in this illegal realm. On ships and on land, health
practitioners participating in the slave trade relied on traditional medical
knowledge as well as on new therapies and methodologies to carry out their
work among slaves and slave traders.

On slave ships they usually carried with them medicine chests and
instructions for how to prepare the necessary remedies to treat the array of
diseases they would be exposed to. Inventories of these medicine chests tell
us what remedies and treatments they were likely to administer and how
effective they might have been. On land, it was a similar situation, as those
in charge of administering the health provision for slave factories frequently
were also able to prepare any needed remedies following written or verbal
instructions.

Medicine chests were a permanent feature on board slave vessels as
well as in slave factories. For example, in 1819, an inventory of medicines
kept at a hospital frequently used by slave traders in Mozambique showed an
extensive selection of drugs to treat some of the most common diseases
found in the slave trade. Among them were the purgative drug jalap; silver
nitrate, which was routinely used to treat ophthalmia; rhubarb, normally
used as a laxative; the popular mercurial drug calomel, employed to fight
fevers and a number of other diseases; emetic tartar, which was convention-
ally used against leichmaniasis and schistosomiasis; *digitalis purpurea* (*tinctura digitalis*), used since the late eighteenth century to treat heart problems;
and camphor and opium, which were also employed to treat a variety of
diseases and illnesses.[93] Likewise, in a list of utensils necessary to provide
medical treatments to those who would use the hospital's services were such
items as glasses of various sizes, spatulas, ivory syringes, and fabrics.[94]

In an analogous list of medicines produced in 1835, at another notorious Portuguese illegal slave-trading haunt, the island of Principe, some of
the same medicines appeared again, including camphor, jalap, emetic tartar,

tinctura digitalis, and opium.[95] Other significant medical remedies and products, like various types of quinine and mercurial drugs, were also present in this list. The presence of quinine in particular confirmed once again the fact that slave traders, just like their nemeses the anti–slave trade patrols, were making heavy use of the extract against fevers, as Captain William Owen had observed during his anti–slave trade mission to the east coast of Africa in the late 1820s and early 1830s. On that occasion Owen noticed that Portuguese residents in Quelimane, most of which were slave traders, rejected treatments "adopted by European surgeons," that they preferred to use Peruvian bark and rhubarb to fight fevers, and that "they never bleed or administer mercury in any type," despite having the lancet and drugs available to them.[96] To the previously mentioned document produced in Principe, a list of required utensils to treat patients—including "black bottles, clay glasses, canteens, and linen bags"—was appended.[97]

Similar lists of medicines were often found on board slave ships journeying to and from the African coast. For example, in 1839, the brigantine *Especulador* was captured by HMS *Electra* and taken to the Court of Mixed Commission of Rio de Janeiro. As court officers conducted an inventory of all items found on board, they discovered a medicine chest that contained, among many other medicines, cardamom, tartar crème, Arabic gum, laudanum, mercury, almond oil, sarsaparilla, ammonia salts, sulfate of quinine, sulfate of magnesium, and pectoral, antiscorbutic, and emollient agents.[98]

A close evaluation of the contents found in these medicine chests, in combination with the stories left behind by slave traders in their private letters and memoirs, allows us to build a picture of the variety and likely effectiveness of the drugs used by slave traders during this period. It is not difficult to conclude that they were aware of the main state-of-the-art drugs and therapies of their time, from the most basic ones, like inoculation or vaccination of African slaves against smallpox, to effective remedies such as quinine-based compounds to fight fevers and ipecacuanha derivatives to treat dysentery.

In addition to the always-necessary medicine chests, slave traders often carried with them meticulous instructions for when and how to use these remedies. On occasion, they also took with them recipes and instructions

that explained, step-by-step, how to prepare healing remedies using the ingredients they had brought on their transatlantic voyages. For example,
among the papers found in 1829 on board the Spanish brig *Segunda Teresa*
were two small pieces of paper giving specific guidelines for curing anyone
affected by smallpox, linking the suggested procedures with the medicines
found in the vessel's medicine chest.[99] Once the symptoms of the disease
had been observed and confirmed, a small dose of emetic "from a little bottle" should be administered after fasting in the morning, or five hours after
every meal. This dose was to be augmented and given more frequently until
the patient had vomited. Only then was a purgative tea to be given in order
to "clean the stomach . . . and the belly."[100]

　　The second piece of paper found on the *Segunda Teresa* concerned
the use of calcium chloride to "cure all types of sores" and to "disinfect and
rarefy the air in any room."[101] To treat sores, the note recommended that the
substance be mixed well in a bottle with water and then applied "using an
ivory syringe, irrigating the sore."[102] As soon as the sore was finally desic-
cated and the raw flesh exposed, a piece of fabric with "the unguent found
in a tin can" should be applied, after which the sore would heal. Calcium
chloride was also recommended as a disinfectant, mixed with water and
sprayed all over a room to disperse bad smells. The note concluded by urg-
ing the captain of the vessel to do this as soon as possible, as such a process
was likely to "avoid many diseases if it was put in place from the beginning
and then kept with perseverance for the rest of the journey."[103]

　　When the French schooner *Aimable Claudine* was captured by a British cruiser in 1825, a medicine chest was found on board. Alongside it were
also two small notes explaining how to prepare and apply some medical
remedies that could be prepared with ingredients obtained from the chest.[104]
One of them was a recipe written in Italian referred to as *lusegetto nero*. The
second one contained instructions to make some of the famous rub of Laffecteur, a popular remedy against syphilis in the first half of the nineteenth
century.[105] After a meticulous description of all the amounts needed from
every root, shrub, and other substances necessary to make the potion, the
note's author suggested boiling them all, with the exception of the sugar
and the honey, which were to be added after the resulting "liqueur" had

been filtered and boiled again for hours. The note, which was probably copied from a book or manual, suggested dosages of four ounces or six spoons for men, three ounces or five spoons for women, and promised that the decoction would cure "venereal diseases" that had been previously treated with mercury—but not gonorrhea.[106]

Perhaps the most exhaustive set of instructions ever produced was given to the master of the Spanish schooner *Magdalena* before he departed on a voyage to West Africa in August 1839. When the vessel was captured by HMS *Viper* in November, while on its way to Gallinas under Portuguese colors, an exhaustive and extensive set of instructions were found on board regarding when and how to use the contents of the ship's medicine chest.[107]

Some of the most interesting prescriptions on this long list concerned the provision of purgatives like the Leroy's elixir, which was to be administered to most patients regardless of their respective ailments, and occasionally in combination with English purgative salts.[108] Tartar crème and castor oil were also recommended as mild purgatives in cases of inflammation of the stomach and other adjacent areas. Liquid laudanum was prescribed to ease pain and help patients to sleep, sometimes in combination with sulfuric ether. Sulfate of quinine, certainly the most effective remedy against malarial fevers, was also extensively described and prescribed. Patients suffering from cold fevers were ordered to take a small dose every two hours, using the index finger and thumb in the same way that tobacco snuff was grabbed to obtain the required amount. It was also suggested that the sulfate of quinine be mixed with chamomile tea for better results.[109]

Other remedies prescribed in this exhaustive set of instructions included some that were widely used at the time, including Emplasto de Andrés de la Cruz, a popular unguent constituted by a mixture of laurel oil, turpentine, and resins, which was prescribed to treat wounds, and Extract of Saturn or Goulard, a lead-and-acetate-based solution that was recommended as an astringent and to treat skin burns and eye diseases like ophthalmia. Also on the list were other prevalent remedies against cough and fever, like Arabic gum; against diarrhea, like tincture of Catecú; and to treat wounds, like Catholic balm.[110]

These thoroughly compiled lists of medicines found on board slave ships and the frequent accompanying instructions for their use reveal to us an underlying world of health practices and medical knowledge that has so far eluded historians of the illegal slave trade. Precisely because of the concealed character of these expeditions, only a small number of exceptionally illustrative documents, mostly preserved thanks to the actions of anti–slave trade officers throughout the Atlantic world, have survived until today. Fortunately, a close reading of their contents allows us to lay bare the resources they had to their disposition in these expeditions as well as to speculate about how knowledgeable those in charge of making remedies out of medicine chest ingredients were.

In a despairing communication sent in 1820 to the Duke of San Fernando, Sierra Leone Mixed Commission judge Francisco Lefer Robaud felt compelled to comment on the effects of lethal diseases not only on the West African British colony but also on slave traders along the coast. He wrote: "On the entire coast there has been much disease. In Rio Pongo there is a vessel that cannot leave because the entire crew has died; and another has lost half of hers."[111] Lefer Robaud's awareness that Spanish sailors were dying in the neighborhood of Sierra Leone was not surprising, as he was probably in constant communication with some of the main slave dealers in the region. This circumstance allowed him to report on a matter that was all too familiar to Spanish slave dealers at the time: the risk for any slave-trading expedition to the coast of Africa of deaths among crew and cargo as a result of the diseases endemic to slave-trade contact zones.

Slave dealers after 1820 repeatedly confronted diseases that threatened not only their human cargoes and their profits but also their own lives. These diseases were present at every stage of the slave trade, and they were unpredictable: in many cases little was known about how they were spread and how they could be contained and treated. Slave vessels were repositories of deadly diseases, where crammed cargoes of human beings suffered from exposure to inclement weather and the notoriously unhealthy environments almost universally found below deck. Slave dealers and any passengers on board of these vessels were continuously exposed to these deadly environments too, as numerous reports of deaths at sea and shortly after arrival at their destinations attest. On these ships, health provision was dispensed by an assortment of practitioners that could range from college-educated medical doctors to mates, boatswains, and cooks. While many of them were white Europeans and Americans, there is evidence too of African and African-descended health practitioners in the illegal slave trade.

Slave factories fared no better. There, slaves were packed in reduced spaces within barracoons, where diseases proliferated. Diseases and famine were common in these factories, particularly in those where anti–slave trade patrol blockades resulted in overcrowding for longer periods of time. Factories along the African coast were quintessential slave-trade contact zones, where Africans and Western traders interacted on a regular basis.

Slave dealers, whether on land or at sea, fought diseases with similar medicinal remedies and treatments as those used by all other Atlantic actors at the time. They consistently used old, traditional therapies and medications, although there is convincing evidence that they also resorted to new treatments and cures as much as those engaged in ending the slave trade did. They regularly depended on medicine chests that contained the ingredients and instructions needed to manufacture the remedies required to fight the diseases they were likely to encounter.

The illegal slave trade was an activity fraught with perils of various kinds, of which diseases were perhaps the most obvious and present. Fighting diseases and limiting their ravages became central on both sides of the Atlantic and at sea. Moreover, slave traders were simultaneously menaced by anti–slave trade patrols and officers across the Atlantic and deadly, debilitating, and incapacitating diseases. The latter were a common enemy shared by all those exposed to the climates of the various African and American regions where the slave trade continued to exist until the second half of the nineteenth century.

Cruising for Slaves and Boating up Rivers

Anti–Slave Trade Patrols and the Fight
against Disease across the Atlantic

We will dance to our graves if we are to die! So here is to ye Messrs Boa
Constrictors, Lions, Tigers, Jackals, Jackasses, Jackanapes, African fever,
and the whole of your damned diabolical, devouring, devastating,
and deplorably detestable crew!
—John C. Lawrence, 1844

IN 1835 GEORGE MCLAREN'S ship, HMS *Serpent,* arrived in the
Caribbean destined to join the West Indies and North American stations
engaged in the suppression of the slave trade. McLaren and the *Serpent*
spent the next few years pursuing slavers, visiting some of the most fascinating places in the region, and struggling against repeated outbreaks of dangerous diseases, often contracted from the same men, women, and children
they were attempting to release, as well as from their captors.

Yellow fever was a frequent subject of reflection in the journal kept by
McLaren during these years. In July 1835, while the ship was anchored at
Port Royal in Jamaica, he referred to it as "that demon Yellow Jack," a disease that usually had "a fatal effect" on those unlucky enough to contract it.[1]
Its devastation among the crew of the *Serpent* was made even clearer when
a few lines later, he felt compelled to mention that scarcely a day passed
without "England's proud banner" being hoisted in memory "of her departed heroes."[2]

McLaren's journal also superbly illustrates the terrible conditions of the Africans found in each of the vessels captured by the *Serpent*. In January 1836, after seizing the *Ninfa Matanzera* with 450 men, women, and children, McLaren commented that by the time the vessel had arrived in Havana, 88 of the slaves originally embarked in Africa had died. Upon inspecting the vessel, he found "the females in a state too horrible to mention."[3] In the following months, McLaren found similarly tragic conditions on board the Spanish brigantine *Empresa* and the Portuguese brigantine *Felix.* The *Empresa,* in particular, was ridden by disease, and according to McLaren, many of the slave dealers apprehended by the *Serpent* "were relieved from fever and other diseases, and owed their very existence to their capture."[4] Not long after, and probably as a result of their contact with these two ships, the *Serpent*'s captain, Evan Nepean, was forced to hoist the yellow flag signaling quarantine just after they reached the island of Grenada.[5]

The experiences of McLaren during his time on the *Serpent* were not very different than those of other crew members, including ship surgeons, throughout the Atlantic. As slave vessels became quintessential slave-trade contact zones, all those involved in stopping them were exposed to the same diseases that slave traders had encountered during their own voyages, as well as any they may have contracted on the ground in Africa while bartering for slaves and loading them onto their ships. Health practitioners were essential for the survival of a ship's own crew, and frequently also for that of slave dealers and the slaves themselves. At sea, where the lack of adequate medical facilities meant that conditions could easily worsen, carrying health practitioners with the necessary expertise, skills, and knowledge to confront deadly diseases was often a matter of life and death.

A Necessary Parenthesis: Western Navies and the Illicit Slave Trade

Soon after the 1807 Slave Trade Abolition Bill was passed by the British Parliament, anti–slave trade patrols began to arrive in West African waters to enforce the new legislation. During the 1810s the British sent a number of cruisers to monitor the area and unilaterally seize slave-trading vessels, while Vice-Admiralty courts were charged with adjudicating cases of vessels considered to be involved in this human traffic. However, not until after the first bilateral treaties were signed with Portugal, Spain, and the Netherlands were proper anti–slave trade squadrons placed in strategic locations on both sides of the Atlantic to pursue and seize vessels from any treaty-signatory nation involved in human trafficking. From early on, the British took it upon themselves to patrol the Atlantic, largely as a response to the lukewarm attitude of other nations. Already in the 1820s, there were British anti–slave trade squadrons along the coasts of Africa and Brazil and in the Caribbean. Slave-trading vessels captured by these cruisers were taken first to the courts of Mixed Commission established in places like Freetown, Rio de Janeiro, and Havana, and within a few years, to courts of Vice-Admiralty located in several locations throughout the Atlantic and the Indian Oceans.[6]

In these early years, two other nations that had originally rejected bilateral treaties with the British granting the mutual right of search of their vessels began to act against the slave trade on both sides of the Atlantic, often combining these efforts, as the British had done, with protocolonialist enterprises.[7] The Americans sent their first ships to the African coast in 1819 and patrolled the area sporadically throughout the 1820s and 1830s, although their main activity in the region was to supply and offer protection to the newly established colony of Liberia.[8] The operations of U.S. ships in Africa had developed almost simultaneously with the creation of two new naval forces: the West Indies and Brazil squadrons. These two squadrons were instituted to repress privateering and piracy in the Caribbean from 1817 onward, and to protect American interests in Brazil from 1826 onward. Both naval forces would eventually evolve into effective anti–slave trade squadrons from the 1840s until the start of the U.S. Civil War, when they were recalled to the United States.[9]

The French, too, began to send armed vessels to Africa in the early 1820s to curb the slave trade carried out by its subjects in the area.[10] Their efforts seem to have been more successful and somewhat more consistent than those of the Americans, although they too were driven by an expansionist agenda. In 1822, for example, British Mixed Commission officers in Sierra Leone informed the foreign secretary that they had seen with their own eyes the arrival of the French armed schooners *Momus* and *Iris* a year earlier, charged with orders of "going down the coast in search of French Slave Traders." In the same letter, the commissioners pointed out that another vessel, the brig *Le Huron,* skippered by the commander of "the French squadron on the coast," had proceeded directly to the Bight of Benin, detained a French vessel, and taken it before the "Judicial Administration of Senegal" for trial.[11]

That same year, the French corvette *La Diane* was also reported to have sailed along West Africa, visiting the coasts of Malaguetta and Gallinas and boarding a number of French vessels suspected "of having the intention of trading in slaves."[12] Some years later, in 1827, the frigate *La Flore* detained the slave vessel *L'Elise* fully fitted for a slave voyage and captained by French aristocrat Dénis de Trobriand. Upon arrival in Gorée, the vessel was condemned, and Trobriand was reprimanded and dismissed as its commander.[13] Two years later, however, he reappeared in Havana, presumably involved in the planning of a new slave-trading expedition to Africa, a circumstance that prompted the French consul in the Cuban capital to write to Paris reporting the entire affair.[14] In these years, the French Navy also intercepted and put to trial a number of vessels at other locations, including Guadeloupe and Cayenne, although their efforts were not always successful.[15]

Throughout the 1820s, most captures of slave vessels were carried out by the British Navy. The courts of Mixed Commission in Sierra Leone, Rio de Janeiro, and Havana processed most of these slave vessels, often adjudicating the cases and condemning the offenders following swift legal hearings. Throughout the 1820s and 1830s the British were at their most effective along the western coast of Africa, although they also captured and adjudicated several vessels carrying slaves (or equipped to do so) on the waters of the West Indies and Brazil, often making substantial sums of money as a reward for each recaptured African they took before the courts of Mixed Commission and later on, of the Vice-Admiralty.[16] In the words of Pedraic X. Scanlan, this "focus on the value of slave ships made the fate of former captives an afterthought."[17]

It was not, however, until the 1840s that concerted efforts carried out by different nations—often coordinated or imposed by the British—began

London, March 17, 1834.

NOTICE is hereby given to the officers and company of His Majesty's sloop Victor, Robert Russell, Esq. Commander, that they will be paid their respective proportions of the bounty granted for slaves captured in the Negrito, on the 21st November 1832, also a moiety of the proceeds of hull, &c. at No. 22, Arundel-street, Strand, on the 10th of April next; where the recalls will be made, agreeably to Act of Parliament.

Flag	-	£302	7	0¼
First class	-	604	14	0½
Second class	-	100	15	8
Third class	-	60	9	4¾
Fourth class	-	16	15	11¼
Fifth class	-	12	17	3
Sixth class	-	9	12	1¼
Seventh class	-	6	8	7½
Eighth class	-	3	4	3¾

Thomas Stilwell *and Sons,* **Agents.**

Fig. 9. Notice to the crew of HMS *Victor. London Gazette,* March 18, 1834.

to yield a larger number of captures and adjudications. The equipment clause in the Anglo-Spanish treaty of 1835, the Palmerston Act of 1839, the repeated attacks on slave factories along the coast of Africa, and the apprehension of some American vessels by British cruisers in the late 1830s all led to significant changes to how the slave trade would be pursued and suppressed in the years to come.[18]

As the British Navy intensified its attempts to capture slave vessels, the U.S. government decided that it was time to send a new anti-slave trade squadron to Africa. Although the squadron's main purpose was to detain U.S. vessels and citizens involved in this traffic, its officers also carried instructions of stop the British from aggressively harassing and boarding U.S. merchant ships against which they had no legal right to move.[19]

By the mid-1840s both the U.S. and French squadrons in West and West Central Africa were in active pursuit of slavers, often in collaboration. Although in several instances conflict arose as a result of the British or the French overstepping their entitlements—notably in the Rio Nuñez affair—the work of the British, American, French, and Portuguese anti-slave trade patrols frequently led to coordinated efforts that yielded a number of captures over the years.

The French squadron had been perhaps one of the most effective in the early part of the 1830s, when its presence along the West African coast all but eliminated the slave traders' habitual practice of using the French ensign to carry out slave-trading voyages. In 1835, Thomas Cole and William Macaulay confessed to Henry John Temple, Viscount Palmerston, that the "activity of the French squadron" had been the main reason behind the destruction of the slave trade "formerly carried out under the French flag."[20] Palmerston himself had been somewhat responsible for this increase of French activities against the slave trade, as he, with the assistance of Viscount Granville, repeatedly pressured French Foreign Minister Count Sébastiani in 1831 to take matters into his hands, reinforcing the French squadron in West Africa.[21] Although French activities were less conspicuous between the mid-1830s and the mid-1840s, from 1845 onward the French became, at least for a while, the main anti–slave trade force at sea in Africa, marshaling as many as twenty-seven vessels in anti–slave trade and protocolonial activities by 1846.[22] This situation led British officers to lament the fact that the French had managed to put together a larger anti–slave trade fleet of vessels than the British themselves, somehow challenging their supremacy and leadership on these waters.[23]

After 1845 the French, who had also had a squadron off the coast of Brazil from the 1830s onward, expanded their operations all along the African coast from their Gorée Island enclave down to the south of Benguela, also with an eye on establishing colonial entrepôts along the coast.[24] Admirals Eduard Bouët-Willaumez and Auguste Baudin had successful stints in charge of the squadron.[25] Baudin was charged with conducting an exploratory mission along the coast with the intention of gathering intelligence on the slave traders and their hideouts, and of finding propitious sites to set up new French enclaves.[26] Simultaneously, another French ship captain and future commander of the squadron, Jérôme Félix de Monleón was tasked with a similar assignment, but he was instructed to pay special attention to the "part of the African littoral, comprising between Cacheo and Seabar."[27]

The French squadron remained in place until the transatlantic slave trade was finally abolished. Its last commander, Andre Emile León Laffon

de Ladebat, abandoned the pursuit of slavers in 1866. During the two decades the French remained active, they frequently collaborated with the
British and on occasion with the Americans and the Portuguese. In June
1846, for example, the steamer *L'Australie*, under the command of Lieutenant La Gallie de Kerirouët, was able to get a supply of coal at Luanda when
its reserves were depleted after capturing a slaver with 275 Africans on
board about ten miles from Loango.[28] The French efforts, like those of the
other squadrons, were frequently recorded and communicated to London
by British officers on land and at sea.[29] Although conflict between the British and the French was rare, matters came to a head in 1849 when two of the
French squadron vessels fired upon two British merchant ships, creating a
protocolonial international diplomatic crisis that came to be known as the
Rio Nuñez affair; the contretemps was not fully resolved until four years
later.[30]

The Portuguese squadron also had its zenith in the second part of the
1840s, especially during the years in which its ships were under the command of commodores Francisco António Gonçalves Cardoso and Manuel
Tomás da Silva Cordeiro. For most of the period the Portuguese squadron
was more concerned with dealing with colonial issues, especially in Benguela, than in carrying out their anti–slave trading duties.[31] According to the
British, the Portuguese squadron captured only a limited number of slave
ships, even during Gonçalves Cardoso's and Cordeiro's years, and their
main successes came whenever they attacked slave factories on the coast.[32]

Collaboration efforts as well as instances of conflict between the Portuguese and the British throughout the 1840s were reported regularly by
British court officers in Luanda and naval officers at sea, as well as by Portuguese officers.[33] In 1848 British and Portuguese cruisers carried out a
joint naval exercise in front of the fortress of Penedo in Luanda, discharging
broadsides and trying a number of naval maneuvers.[34] In 1849, Commodore
Charles Hotham detailed at length his efforts to persuade his Portuguese
counterpart to attack and destroy the slave barracoons at Mazula and Ambriz.[35] According to Hotham, when he offered to help in this task, the Portuguese Commodore declined, replying that he was not allowed to carry
out joint operations with the British. Soon after this conversation took

place, the *Mondego* sailed alone from Luanda toward these two sites on the coast and proceeded to destroy them by sending the boats of the vessel against them. Two years later, Hotham's successor, Commodore Arthur Fanshawe, echoed his colleague's opinion of Cordeiro and the Portuguese squadron, pointing out that their work together had been "very cordial," and that they had developed a mutual "good understanding" during their "friendly intercourse."[36] As a matter of fact, more than once Gonçalves Cardoso and Cordeiro ran into difficulties with their own government for openly liaising with the British. Eventually, and in spite of British protestations, Captain Graça, with whom the British would never achieve a similar level of collaboration, replaced Cordeiro in 1851.[37]

The British developed a closer rapport with the U.S. squadron. Even though the British repeatedly created potential diplomatic issues by boarding American vessels, these situations were consistently defused, and the navies' collaborative work continued until the U.S. Civil War began in 1861, when all American vessels were recalled.[38] The collaborative efforts between the British and American squadrons on occasion led to the capture of slavers, and were widely praised by both governments. In one such instance, Captain J. S. Nicholas of the U.S. Navy and Commander Norman B. Bedingfield of the Royal Navy undertook a series of operations together in the spring of 1861, leading to the capture of the American ship *Triton*, found fully equipped for the slave trade, by USS *Constellation* on the Congo River, and the destruction of the Spanish schooner *Jacinta*, by the boats of the steamer HMS *Prometheus*. The story of these two seizures was blown out of proportion by both governments, becoming the subject of mutual praise between Richard Bickerton Pemell, Viscount Lyons, the British Ambassador to the United States, and Secretary of State William H. Seward, each praising the importance of the other navy's help.[39]

From the mid-1840s until their recall in the summer of 1861, U.S. ships posted along the African coast made thirty-six captures, which, added to those made between 1845 and 1849 off the Brazilian coast, and those made between 1858 and 1860 off Cuba, amounted to a total of fifty-one vessels interdicted for their involvement on the slave trade.[40] However, irrespective of the level of engagement of the U.S. squadrons on both sides of

the Atlantic, or the size of the French squadron in the 1840s, none ever really rivaled the British in effectiveness, commitment, and aggressiveness—
even during those periods in which their actions were severely compromised
and their effectiveness strictly limited.

In fact, quite often the British were alone in their efforts to bring the
slave trade to an end. This was particularly the case whenever they had to
rely on the voluntary cooperation of corrupt authorities, often themselves
involved in the traffic, as it was the case with the colonial and imperial officers in Havana, Salvador de Bahia, and Rio de Janeiro. In Havana, for example, the British squadron was repeatedly led away from the slave traders
by virtually anyone with a position of authority in the island—including
most of the captains general of the period. Years after abandoning his post,
former Captain General Miguel Tacón recalled in detail that during his time
in Havana he had done everything in his power to assist the slave traders
and deceive the British Navy and the Mixed Commission officers and consuls living in the island. In his own words, during his governorship of Cuba
(1834–38):

> Every time the English Commissioners denounced before the
> Captain General the arrival of one of them [slave vessels] to one
> of the [Cuba's] ports, after landing their blacks, the denounce-
> ment was passed along to the Marine department where an in-
> vestigation always favorable to the accused was to be launched,
> as the captains' log books and the depositions of those who had
> arrived in those ships, always proved the accusations to be
> unfounded.[41]

In Brazil practices were no different. There, preparations for illegal
expeditions to Africa and concealed landings continued to take place in
spite of the pressure applied by the British. The British consul in Bahia remarked in a letter to Foreign Minister George Canning in 1827 that the Ba-
hian government suffered from "perverse blindness and diseased optics."[42]
In the words of Brazilian historian Luis Viana Filho, the Brazilians had
decided to apply a policy of "neither seeing nor hearing" evidence of the

slave trade, just as their Cuban counterparts were doing.[43] This situation did not change until even heavier pressures from the British in the mid- to late 1840s forced the Brazilians finally to agree to the final abolition of slave traffic.[44]

By the late 1830s, such malfeasance inspired British Foreign Minister Viscount Palmerston to begin a new push against the slave trade. The modifications in the modus operandi of slave traders after the Anglo-Spanish treaty of 1835's equipment clause was signed were central to the implementation of these new strategies. The resulting Palmerston Act of 1839 was mostly concerned with addressing these new stratagems, particularly the abuse of the Portuguese flag in order to avoid capture, and its consequences were immediately felt across the Atlantic world.[45]

The Palmerston Act empowered British anti–slave trade squadrons to carry out more daring expeditions against slave factories—as in fact they did—but also to stop and search any Portuguese vessel and, more important, any flagless vessel. The captured ships were then taken to courts of Vice-Admiralty located in a series of Atlantic ports—plus one in an Indian Ocean port at the island of Mauritius—where cases were swiftly adjudicated without the hassle that had plagued the courts of Mixed Commissions' two-party system for years, and where the Africans found on board were often given care and subsequently emancipated.

Whether in Africa, Brazil, or the Caribbean, captures of slavers, destruction of barracoons, and emancipation of Africans were all part of the work of every British Navy ship assigned to anti–slave trade duties. Their operations were frequently fraught with dangers of various kinds, from deadly diseases to violent resistance by the slave traders, but the crews were also handsomely remunerated with monetary rewards and promotions. Over the years, and in spite of their limited success and secondary motivations, they chipped away at human trafficking in the Atlantic and rescued thousands of men, women, and children from the hands of unscrupulous slave dealers, while also strengthening formal and informal British imperialist endeavors in these regions. By means of their routine contact with local populations, they also learned about the diseases of the slave trade and the best ways to prevent and treat them.

Chasing and Seizing Slavers

The pursuing of slave vessels was in many ways a perilous enterprise. Over the years, ships and crews involved in executing abolitionist policies throughout the Atlantic were subjected to the inclemency of the various Atlantic climates, to the regular actions of resistance presented by the slave traders, and to the microbes with which they cohabited the contact zones of the slave trade on both sides of the Atlantic. Although anti–slave trade patrols, prize officers, and health practitioners all profited from every captured vessel and every recaptured African, they often considered relocation to these regions as a death sentence.[46] Fear and anxiety, then, were prevalent among them, especially in years like 1823, 1829–30, 1837, and 1847, when epidemics of yellow fever raged across European settlements along the coast, and on several of the vessels attached to these squadrons.

The 1829–30 season in particular seems to have had a deep impact on all those involved in the anti–slave trade efforts along the African coast, and even in the Caribbean. Captain William Owen, one of the stalwarts of the British anti–slave trade naval forces in the region at the time, commented in his memoirs about the state of mind of his crew, pointing out that the "constant operation of committing their companions to the deep, and a superstitious fancy that they were going to be the next victims, preyed upon and depressed the spirits of the men."[47] In his opinion, the real impact of these diseases was much more "the result of fear and anticipation than of the climate."[48]

Peter Leonard, while recounting his experiences among the sailors of the West African squadron, also referred to the usual fears of death among the crew of HMS *Plumper,* while contrasting them with its normalization on land, where, in his words, death was "a matter of such common occurrence, that the subject is seldom spoken of on shore." Leonard also examined the ways in which sailors coped with these fears and anxieties by narrating how some of them would "make a few jokes" about the real possibility of their own deaths.[49] He went on to point out, almost in a stoic fashion, that "jesting in this manner with the risk [they] run disarms it of half its terrors."[50]

Highly apprehensive and stressed officers and crews seem to have been the norm then, at least after the slave trade became illicit across the

Atlantic basin from the 1820s onward. To the crews from British, French, American, and other nations' vessels, patrolling large geographical areas was at once a blessing and a curse. In an illustrative case, the surgeon of the Portuguese brig *Audaz,* engaged in the abolition of the slave trade along the Angolan coast, reported in 1841 that one of the officers traveling on his vessel developed a sudden "monomania," first trying to commit suicide by jumping into the sea, and then becoming aggressive toward the rest of the crew, until he was finally subdued and taken to a hospital in Luanda.[51]

Even the knowledge of an upcoming appointment to the African station could be a source of anxiety and uneasiness. James Dick, a surgeon with the British Navy from the early 1850s onward, confessed to having been aghast upon finding in 1862 that he had been attached to HMS *Flying Fish,* a vessel that was about to join the West African squadron. Dick "tried to get off the appointment" without success, and was left with little else to do than stoically trying to make "the best of a bad bargain."[52]

Having the opportunity to escape particularly morbid areas was definitely an advantage that anti–slave trade patrol vessels repeatedly benefited from. Just as the French would retire to the relatively healthy climate of the island of Gorée, the British were able to choose among various locations that included the islands of Ascension and Saint Helena, as well as the Cape of Good Hope. The downside of laboring in such a vast realm was that sailors frequently spent extensive periods of time at sea, and not uncommonly they did so while most or many were struggling against fevers and other diseases, or recovering from their ravages.

For example, vessels from various nations attached to their respective West African squadrons often had to patrol entire geographical regions as extensive as the West African coast from the Senegambia to the Bight of Biafra and the Cameroon River, or from Cape Lopez to Benguela and Little Fish Bay. On the other side of the ocean, the multiple geographical features of the Brazilian coast, and the numerous isles and keys scattered throughout the Caribbean Sea, made their anti–slave trade patrols extremely arduous, as they presented slave traders with perfect routes and endless possibilities to evade and escape capture.[53]

Along the African coast, forced by the new hostile policies of Britain and other nations, slave traders began to move away from the coastline and into the interior of rivers and other waterways. By 1830, there were few slave factories along the coastline of Upper Guinea, and most of those that could be found on the rivers Gallinas, Sestos, and Pongo were all now located inland, often in the labyrinths formed by mangrove marshes and swamps, where anti–slave trade patrol boats could get easily lost and come back empty-handed. Along the Bight of Benin the situation was similar, as most established factories and slave-trading posts, such as Jakin, Ouidah, Badagry, and Onim, were by the inland lagoon and not on the actual coast. Likewise, most of the factories on the Bight of Biafra, the Cameroon River, Cape Lopez, and the Congo delta, were moved inland to avoid being easily seen by the anti–slave trade cruisers and their boats.

To add to their woes, severely inclement weather, including the harmattan winds and tropical storms often referred to as tornadoes, could make the pursuit and capture of slave expeditions all the more demanding. In the Caribbean, the tropical hurricane season, running from June to November, also constituted a yearly reminder of the perils associated with the enforcement of anti–slave trade policies on the Atlantic. Reports on shipwrecks and crews and vessels lost at sea were common during the period, dire reminders of the dangers associated with these activities.

At sea and on land, stalking and pursuing slave traders called for bravery, endurance, diplomacy, and intelligence. As the nineteenth century wore on and anti-slavery patrols became more visible, slave traders became more and more cunning in response, and they employed all available resources to flee from their pursuers.[54] Thus, anti–slave trade patrols not only had to be able to spot, give chase, and board slave vessels—which were often faster and better armed—but once on board, they had to be able to negotiate their way around false papers and flags, foreign accents, and other schemes for deception.

These same skills—endurance, diplomacy, and intelligence—were absolutely necessary for those officers and sailors who were forced to abandon the relative safety of their vessels and go on shore, whether in boating expeditions against slave dealers, to replenish their provisions, or to carry out

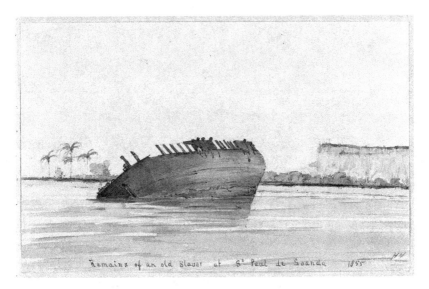

Fig. 10. Slaver shipwreck at Luanda. NMM: Album. Art/10. MS65/134.

negotiations with local rulers on the African coast and with corrupt and conniving authorities in places like Brazil and Cuba. Negotiations with local rulers became more and more common after the 1830s, when the British began imposing bilateral treaties on many coastal rulers and states in exchange for trading concessions or through the use of veiled, and sometimes not-so-veiled, military threats.

Carrying out these negotiations necessarily involved visits on shore, and on occasion these could last for days or weeks at a time. The letters of commander Hugh Dunlop to his sister Fanny and other relatives in the late 1840s are a testament to these perils. Dunlop was credited with bringing the slave trade to an end on the infamous river Gallinas when he engaged in protracted negotiations with the local rulers, which resulted in these chiefs banishing the slave trade and surrendering to him nearly fifteen hundred slaves and fifty-five slave dealers. In these letters, Dunlop reported to his sister that in order to complete this negotiation he had been forced to go on shore on three occasions, the first time for a period of sixteen days, the second for ten days, and the final time for eighteen days. He confessed to her that he had been attacked by the fever during each of his expeditions,

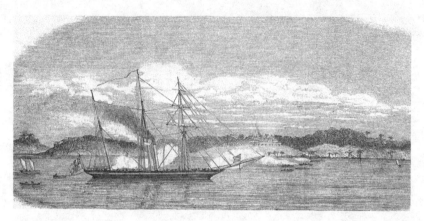

Fig. 11. HMS *Teazer* attacking Medina. *Illustrated London News,* May 14, 1853.

reflecting that unfortunately he "could not have done what has been done without going on shore."[55] It is worth noticing that in these missions Dunlop relied mostly on the Kroomen he had with him on HMS *Alert,* "being afraid to expose [his officers] to that vile climate at the very worst season."[56]

A more graphic narrative of a similar process of negotiation was given by Captain Henry Need, commander of HMS *Linnet,* while on duty on the West African station between 1852 and 1854. Soon after arriving at his destination, Commander Need, accompanied by Lieutenant Rich of HMS *Teazer,* was dispatched to the town of Medina, not far from the British colony of Sierra Leone. Their mission was to request that the town honor the treaty it had previously signed with the British, banning the slave trade, and that it surrender a British man whom townspeople had kidnapped from Sierra Leone. When the town's leader, Kaleh Modoo, refused to give up the British subject, Commander Need turned the guns of the *Linnet* and the *Teazer* on the small town and after shelling it for just under one hour, he returned, taking chief Modoo prisoner until the British subject was finally released.[57]

The visual depictions of the entire incident by Commander Need, who was an able artist, combined with the correspondence and newspaper news that followed, constitute an exceptional report of an early show of strength of British gunboat imperialism in the region. Commander Need's

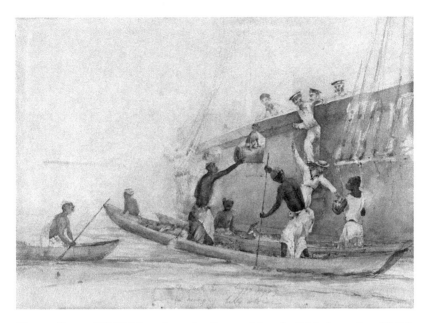

Fig. 12. Crew of HMS *Linnet* bartering for provisions in Cabinda, c. 1853. NMM: Album. Art/10. MS65/134.

watercolors, however, also revealed his communications with local rulers in other parts of Africa, and the ways in which the crew of an anti–slave trade patrol, including the always-present Kroomen, would normally interact with West African populations while in search for slaves, or when in need of supplies. In his watercolors it is possible to see how bartering for products was often done, with locals coming on canoes to the sides of the vessel to exchange their produce—which in some of the drawings include also such animals as monkeys, pigs, and goats—for merchandise.

Medical remedies seem to have been central to these negotiations. In one specific case, while visiting Crawford Island in search of fresh produce and food, Mr. Thornton, a liberated African settled there, wrote to inform Commander Need that in addition to a sheep he had sold to his Kroomen, his wife had sent a bottle of pepper, some cassava, and a plant known as syncongy, almost certainly *Costus dubius,* which was "highly valued amongst the natives on account of its medicinal qualities."[58]

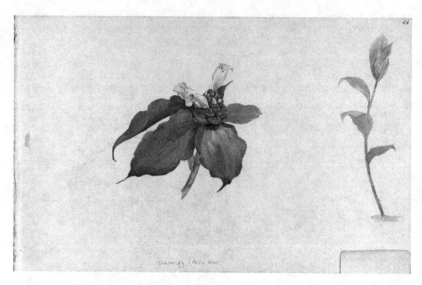

Fig. 13. Syncongy. NMM: Album. Art/10. MS65/134.

Commander Need also illustrated boating expeditions sent on shore and up rivers to pursue and surprise slave dealers. His watercolors complement the narratives of several officers and sailors who left descriptions of the perils associated with what was universally considered the most dangerous job undertaken by anti–slave trade patrol crews. Such expeditions faced the probability that slave dealers would fight back upon being discovered; the always-present dangers of the West African surf; and the threat of catching the dreaded African fevers from going on shore, especially while traveling up rivers. Riverboat expeditions also faced fearsome local predators, including sharks, alligators, hippopotamuses, and large felines. James Dick was one of those who took time to discuss at some length these dangers, commenting in April 1862 that "alligators, some of them of a large size are found, as well as sharks in this river [Nuñez]."[59] Dick went on to describe a twelve-hour "alligator-shooting" expedition up the same river, undertaken by him and some of his mates a couple of days later.[60]

References to these risks and fears were common in the letters sent to Europe and the United States by the officers of the anti–slave trade squadron vessels. Augustus Arkwright, who unlike many others volunteered to the West African squadron in the hope of having a rapid rise within the ranks in the British Navy, commented that "boating up rivers" was "an employment attended with every disadvantage, except the chance of promotion."[61] While recollecting his own experience in West Africa, John C. Lawrence of the United States' African squadron also reflected on the fact that surprising slave dealers at work on the rivers of Upper Guinea "required picking his way through the shoals and flats at the river's mouth, then going upriver. [Commander] Bell knew the risk of exposure to disease was great, but his orders were explicit."[62] Lawrence's opinion was shared by French naval officer Ernest de Cornulier, who was engaged in similar activities while serving the French West African squadron in the early 1820s. De Cornulier commented in his journal that "the more one advances upriver, the more common and dangerous the diseases are."[63]

Alexander Bryson, perhaps better than anyone else, articulated the fears and anxieties associated with going on shore and upriver when he commented in his 1847 book that based on the existing records, it was "apparent that fevers were more likely to attack those who had gone on boat expeditions to the various rivers along the coast."[64] Later on, and basing his reasoning on the experience of the boats of HMS *Owen Glendower* in the rivers of the Bight of Biafra, he went on to squarely blame the boat service carried out by the Royal Navy along the coast and especially on the rivers as the main culprit for the spread of diseases among the crews.[65]

There is little doubt that visits to the coast certainly exposed crews of anti–slave trade patrols to the many diseases endemic in each of these regions. In April 1839, Vicente José dos Santos Moreira Lima, commander of the Portuguese brig *Audaz*, confessed in a letter that his men "had suffered many fevers" and that they were "still suffering" after going on shore. Among those who had perished were two cabin boys and the ship's boatswain.[66]

Several months later Francisco António Gonçalves Cardoso also referred to the fevers that had attacked his crew on the Portuguese ship *Tejo*, complaining about the untimely deaths of his carpenter and caulker, two of the most important members of the crew.[67] The following year, Gonçalves Cardoso was still mourning their deaths and lamenting the "terrible ravages" caused by the fevers on all the ships of the Portuguese anti–slave trade

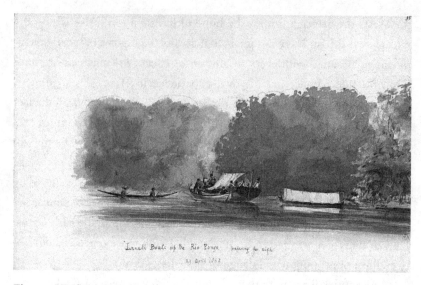

Fig. 14. HMS *Linnet*'s boats preparing to spend the night up the river Pongo, c. 1853. NMM: Album. Art/10. MS65/134.

squadron in Africa.[68] Captain Owen of the British Navy also had some extraordinary observations to make after a visit to the Maputo River in the early 1830s. In this narrative, Owen was perhaps the first person ever, at least in Africa, to link the morbidity of the coast and rivers, and in particular its lethal fevers, with the prevalence of mosquitos, going so far as to suggest that they could be responsible for the fevers suffered by his men:

> The musquitoes were so numerous on board, and indeed everywhere, that it was absolutely impossible to obtain any rest night or day. . . . Every thing was tried, but in vain; the poison of their bite sets the blood in a ferment, and a single mosquito would in many subjects produce a fester accompanied with much pain and fever. . . . To this cause may certainly be attributed much of the mortality that attended this complaint, but whether originating or aggravating the disease is a question not so easily determined. In the course of our experience, the first attacked with the fever were always those who had suffered most from the musquitoes.[69]

Perhaps the most dangerous operations carried out by anti-slavery patrols were their customary attacks on slave-trading ships and the destruction of barracoons, which also involved visits to the coast and often going up the rivers. The destruction of barracoons in particular was fraught with violent hazards that included the possible resistance not only of slave dealers but also of the local rulers who were often their allies and partners. These attacks became more frequent after the famous destruction of the Gallinas factory of Pedro Blanco by a British force led by Captain Joseph Denman in 1840. That year, after finding out about the kidnapping of two British subjects who were being held there, the governor of Sierra Leone, Richard Doherty ordered Denman to sail for Gallinas and rescue them.[70]

Denman duly took the British ships HMS *Wanderer,* HMS *Rolla,* and HMS *Saracen* to Gallinas, crossed the sandbar, and entered the river. After Manna, the son of local ruler Siaka, ignored Denman's attempt to negotiate the captives' release by diplomatic means, the British captain burned down the barracoons and freed the slaves. Denman eventually forced Manna to sign a treaty surrendering all the slaves and the slave traders under his protection. All in all, Denman rescued 841 Africans from the barracoons. Viscount Palmerston, upon being told about the success of Denman's expedition, was said to have exclaimed, "Taking a wasp's nest . . . is more effective that catching the wasps one by one."[71]

Two years later, this time under the command of Captain Joseph Foote, two of the South Atlantic Station vessels, HMS *Madagascar* and HMS *Waterwitch* headed for the slave ports of Cabinda and Ambriz and did the same there, destroying the barracoons and taking with them a large number of Africans to Saint Helena. The *Waterwitch,* under the command of Captain Henry Matson, arrived in Jamestown on June 3, 1842, with 465 Africans on board. The *Madagascar,* under the orders of Captain Foote, reported to be carrying between 200 and 300 more, arrived soon afterward.[72] This effective operation raised expectations about further diminishing the slave trade in the area. Christopher Vowell, the surgeon in charge of the Africans taken to Saint Helena, commented that the destruction of these barracoons would "doubtless give a heavy blow to the trade for the present."[73] Matson himself recounted years later that around 1842 the slave trade had "almost ceased," thanks to the many treaties enforced on local African chiefs, allowing the squadron to destroy any barracoons they could find in those territories.[74] According to Matson the trade restarted within a short period of time due to a letter written by the Earl of Aberdeen in May 1842 in which he questioned the legality of such attacks on the slave barracoons, and to the publicity given to the trial of Joseph Denman in London, which was said to have emboldened slave traders along the African coast.[75]

Regardless, new attacks on slave factories along the coast were carried out in the following years, not just by the British but also by the French and the Portuguese. In 1845, French Commander Auguste Baudin again attacked the factories at Gallinas. Finding them deserted upon his arrival, he complained that the slavers had been warned about his approach and had subsequently headed for the interior with all the slaves they had at the barracoons.[76] The Portuguese too, particularly during the tenure of Commodore Cordeiro in the late 1840s and early 1850s, appear to have been quite active in attacking slave factories in West Central Africa. They were reported to have destroyed the barracoons of Ambriz and Mazula in 1849 and to have burned "a few huts along the coast" in 1851.[77]

Even after the Earl of Aberdeen deemed these excursions as violations of the Laws of Nations and existing bilateral treaties, the British continued to attack and destroy slave factories whenever one of their subjects was kidnapped and sold as a slave in one of them. A case in question was the new attack on the Gallinas River barracoons in 1845 by a British force under the command of Commodore William Jones. After discovering that two British subjects who had been kidnapped were being kept in irons at the factory of Spanish dealer Andrés Jiménez in Dombocorro, Jones first attempted to negotiate a peaceful outcome with Prince Manna, but seeing that his efforts were being wasted, he resorted to gunboat diplomacy instead.[78] On February 4, 1845, Jones "entered the river Gallinas with 286 men, in 18 boats, from Her Majesty's ships Penelope, Growler, and Larne." While Commander Buckle occupied Dombocorro, the rest of the force took up "position in front of Tindes."[79] Eventually, and after more attempts to negotiate led nowhere, a frustrated Jones ordered the total destruction of Tindes, which was "speedily reduced to ashes." Soon after Taillah and

Minnah were also "burnt to the ground." Later the force also went to Seabar, where it proceeded to destroy the barracoons at Boom Kittum.[80]

In East Africa, too, British anti-slavery vessels, occasionally in tandem with their Portuguese counterparts, attacked and destroyed slave factories along the coast. In November 1845, for example, Commander R. B. Crawford of the British Navy and Captain Pedro Valente da Costa Pinho of the Portuguese Navy carried out a joint operation against the slave traders at Pomba Bay.[81] Attacks like this one were also reported in the pages of British newspapers and magazines, occasionally accompanied by graphic depictions of the burning and destruction of the slave barracoons, as in the case of a report on the slave trade in the Mozambique channel, published by the *Illustrated London News* in January 1851.[82]

At sea, violent encounters with slave traders were not infrequent. The speed of slave-trade ships, especially U.S.-built clippers, became a weapon to avoid capture. Some of these clippers were so fast and appropriate for the slave trade that once taken by British cruisers, they were turned into anti–slave trade patrol vessels, perhaps the most famous case being the Brazilian slaver *Henriquetta*, a Baltimore-built schooner captured and rechristened HMS *Black Joke*, which went on to capture several slave-trading vessels.[83]

Many of these ships, including the *Prince of Guinea*, also captured in 1826, and especially commissioned to Philadelphia-based contractor James D. Pratt by Francisco Félix de Souza, often offered stern resistance to the cruisers of the anti-slavery patrols that attempted to stop and search them.[84] When confronted by HMS *Hope*, the *Prince of Guinea* resisted, first using its speed in an attempt to escape—the chase lasted twenty-eight hours— then fighting desperately for two hours and forty minutes.[85]

Resistance to anti-slavery patrols was common and sometimes lethal to all involved. Two notorious cases that took place in the Caribbean in the span of a week in 1829 illustrate the dangers associated with boarding—or attempting to board—and detaining slave ships. On June 22, 1829, HMS *Pickle*, under the command of Lieutenant J. B. B. MacHardy, gave chase to a vessel that appeared to be a fast slaver and turned out to be the Spanish brig *Voladora*. As the pursuit came to a close and the British man-of-war approached the ship, the slaver's captain and crew, "confident of their superior force," bore down on the *Pickle* and attacked the British ship.[86] The action lasted for one hour and twenty minutes, and by the end, the *Voladora* was forced to surrender, having been wrecked by the broadsides of the *Pickle*. Two British sailors perished in the action, and eight more were wounded, some of them seriously. On the *Voladora*'s side, at least fourteen were killed in the attack, and other deaths probably went unreported. According to William Macleay, judge of the court of Mixed Commission in Havana, the risks undertaken by Lieutenant Hardy and his men were consistent with having taken on a vessel three times the size of the *Pickle*, much better armed, and with a much larger crew.[87]

Barely five days later a similar encounter took place between the Spanish brig *Midas* and the smallest ship of war in the entire British Navy, HMS *Monkey*, at the time under the command of Lieutenant Joseph Sherer. In trying this case, Macleay again went to great lengths to explain that the *Midas* was a much larger ship than the *Monkey*—at least four times as large— and that it was well prepared for armed confrontation against any British man-of-war.[88] Although this encounter was less costly to the British, the slavers lost several men, including their first mate, and a number of enslaved Africans who were forced to take arms to fight against the British.

Over the following years similar actions recurred throughout the Atlantic, as well as in the Indian Ocean near the East African coast. Some of the most notorious confrontations took place in West African waters. Among these were the attack on the *Veloz Pasajera* in 1830, which resulted in three British sailors being killed, and several, including the captain, wounded.[89] Even more remarkable was the case of the Spanish brig *Formidable*, captured on December 17, 1834, by HMS *Buzzard*, under the command of Lieutenant Anthony William Milward. The *Formidable* was a large vessel, heavily armed and crewed by sixty-six men. According to Thomas Cole and William Macaulay, who reported on the case from Freetown, "the order, discipline, and regularity, observed in the management of the vessel, giving her so much the appearance of a brig-of-war, which she formerly was; all combined to make her the subject of continual remark, and it was expected that she would not quietly submit to capture, should she be fallen in with by one of the smaller cruizers on this station."[90] After what was described as "an spirited resistance," the *Formidable* finally yielded to the *Buzzard,* not before wounding several British sailors, losing six of its own men, and having sixteen wounded.[91]

Even after captured ships were under full control, various hazards continued to threaten British sailors. Resistance was still a problem, as many prize crews found out during the period, as were piracy, the climate, and even the same slaves they had come to rescue, who were often suffering from a wide range of diseases. Piracy in particular was an always-present concern for anti–slave trade patrols, and especially for prize crews who were in charge of directing seized vessels to port for trial.

Reports of mutinies on board seized vessels or prize vessels being attacked and retaken by slave dealers were not rare, and on occasion British officers were forced to admit that some ships and prize crews had probably been lost to the same slave traders they had taken prisoners. For example, in 1826, Havana Mixed Commission judges Henry Theo Kilbee and William Macleay informed Foreign Minister George Canning that they had received intelligence from the French consul in nearby Santiago de Cuba, a Monsieur Dannery, regarding a Spanish vessel that had entered that port with two recaptured unnamed ships that allegedly had been seized by the British off the coast of Africa. According to the French consul, Kilbee and Macleay reported, the British prize crews "had been murdered by the Spaniards."[92]

In one of the best-documented cases of this kind, members of the crews of the slave-trading ships *Felicidade* and *Echo* joined forces in 1845 to retake the former vessel after they realized that the prize officer and crew were poorly armed and susceptible to defeat. The *Felicidade* had been captured by HMS *Wasp* off the coast of Africa in late February 1845, fully fitted for a slave-trading voyage. Soon after seizing the ship Lieutenant Stoppard gave chase to another slave ship, the *Echo,* which he also captured and found to be carrying more than four hundred African slaves. Seeing himself isolated from the *Wasp,* and with limited resources and men, he decided to take over the *Echo* in order to feed and provide care for the Africans, while leaving Midshipman Thomas Palmer and five other sailors in charge of the *Felicidade,* where most of the slave crews were also placed. Soon the slavers rose, murdered all the British sailors, took over the *Felicidade,* and even attempted to recapture the *Echo,* fleeing when they realized that their chances of doing so were slim. The *Felicidade* sailed away only to be captured again days later by HMS *Star.* The slave traders/mutineers/pirates were then sent to England, where they were put to trial at the Exeter Crown Court, a circumstance that made their story well known, unlike the many others that remained anonymous to posterity.

While seizing slave vessels, another concern for anti–slave trade officers and crews were the very Africans they were attempting to carry away to a safe destiny. In addition to the potentially deadly infectious diseases they often carried, African resistance to anti–slave trade patrols was always a possibility. For example, consider the case of the *Aventuera* or *Ventura,* captured early in 1850 off the coast of Angola with 455 African slaves by HMS *Cyclops,* captained by George Fowler Hastings.

After the vessel was taken, Captain Hastings sent Lieutenant A. B. Hodgkinson and a number of sailors to take over the ship and direct it toward Saint Helena, where its case was to be heard by the Court of Vice-Admiralty. According to the subsequent report, while on the passage to Saint Helena, the Africans, almost certainly spurred by the Brazilian cook of the *Aventuera,* Palma, who knew their language, rose against the prize crew. The Africans wounded some of the crew, but soon found themselves overpowered and facing defeat.[93] Many of them retreated to the hold of the ship, but others jumped overboard, resulting in five deaths; many more would have died but for the efforts of the prize crew, who rescued many more from the ocean just as they were about to perish. Hodgkinson suggested that although the main reason for the Africans to take arms was their "ardent desire to return to their own country," Palma was the main culprit, as he had led them to believe that "they would be taken to a distant part of the world, and there ill-treated; and also that it was doubtful if the water would last the voyage."[94]

All in all, chasing and seizing a slave vessel was an activity fraught with dangers that did not end with the capture. In fact, boarding and taking command of these vessels, which were frequently unseaworthy and packed with large groups of suffering men, women, and children, presented challenges, many of them medical and epidemiological, that needed to be addressed from the moment anti–slave trade officers and crews took command.

Fighting Disease on Seized Slave Ships

Once slave vessels were seized by anti–slave trade patrol cruisers, a number of actions were needed to secure the crew and the Africans on board in order to avoid instances such as the ones that took place on the *Felicidade,* the *Echo,* and the *Aventuera* from occurring. Both crewmen and the enslaved Africans were frequently found suffering from numerous diseases. For prize officers, prize crews, and surgeons in charge of captured slave vessels, managing the ravages of these diseases became perhaps the single most important issue to be attended to.

All parties involved were well aware that they were exposed to these diseases from the moment they boarded the vessels. In 1829 Thomas Butter found himself at Ascension Island and about to return to England from his assignment in the West African squadron when a deadly yellow fever epidemic broke out among a number of British ships of the squadron while they were anchored at Fernando Po. As a result, Butter was ordered to replace the deceased assistant surgeon in one of those ships, HMS *Sybille,* where twenty-four men had perished in a short period of time, and where many were still fighting for their lives. As the vessel made its way south to Saint Helena, the fever ceased and the crew recovered almost completely. However, almost as soon as normality had been reestablished, the *Sybille* captured a slave ship carrying 387 Africans. As a direct result, Butter noted, "a few days afterwards the fever broke out" again, and conditions worsened further soon after, when the *Sybille* seized yet another slaver with 319 Africans.[95] Eventually, "the fever increased to such a degree" that the captain of the *Sybille* had no option but to stop the ship's patrolling duties and to sail again for the healthier climate of Saint Helena.[96] In spite of this course of action, this time the fever took a long time to disappear, and several of the crew were lost to it.

Countless cases recorded by British, French, and American anti–slave trade patrols corroborate the dangers associated with the boarding and taking over of slave ships, and the likely effects that the diseases carried by those slaves and crews could have among their own men. For example, in 1840, William Gore Ouseley, British consul in Rio de Janeiro, observed that diseases carried by the Africans could affect prize officers and crews, citing the case of Lieutenant Albert Haseltine, who while assigned to HMS *Electra* had "caught an infection of a dangerous species of small-pox, and [who] was for some months ill"; Ouseley added that other officers had suffered from the same disease at the time.[97] Equally, taking possession of slave vessels full of sick Africans frequently led to extreme tiredness and angst among prize officers and crews. S. Richardson, a midshipman on HMS *Maidstone* in the mid-1820s, confessed in a private letter that after being put in charge of a captured vessel with 174 Africans in the Bight of Benin, where deaths "occurred daily," he was frequently "ill from the fatigue and anxiety on the passage" to Sierra Leone.[98] In a similar instance, in January 1836 Rear Admiral Sir Graham Eden Hammond begged the judges of the Mixed Commission Court at Rio de Janeiro to disembark as soon as possible all the Africans who had been taken there by a prize crew on board the brig *Orion,* in order "to relieve the officers and men hitherto in charge of her, from the anxious and disgusting duty, as speedily as possible."[99]

One of the best-documented cases on the best ways of dealing with the hazards presented by captured vessels full of moribund slaves was left by the surgeon and assistant surgeon of HMS *Cleopatra,* after their vessel captured the Spanish ship *Progresso,* with 447 slaves aboard, off the coast of Quelimane. Even though the slaves had been embarked only the day before capture, they were found in such a dreadful state of health that James Kittle, the *Cleopatra*'s surgeon, called them "the most wretched beings [he] had ever seen in a slave vessel during [his] five years' service on the coast of Africa."[100] The Africans were suffering from some common diseases found in slave vessels, including dysentery, fevers, craw craw, and skin ulcers, many of which presented a potential risk of contagion to the crew of the *Cleopatra.*

Kittle and his assistant surgeon, Henry Piers, boarded the ship as soon as it was seized and set out to treat the sick Africans, most of whom were children or young adolescents, to the best of their capabilities and knowledge. Seeing the terrible conditions in which the young men and women had been crowded together, Captain Christopher Wyvill ordered Kittle to transfer a number of the Africans to the *Cleopatra* in order to mitigate their suffering. This order created an immediate conflict between the captain and his medical officers, who considered it ill-advised, as "the risk of endangering the ship's company with the existing diseases amongst the negroes" was too high.[101] The disagreement between the captain and the surgeons was eventually resolved a few days later, when they agreed on a new plan presented by the captain, in which he proposed to carefully select fifty of the healthiest Africans to move to the pinnace of the *Cleopatra,* where they could be kept separated from the rest of the British crew.[102]

The notes of Assistant Surgeon Piers on the situation on board the *Progresso* and the administration of medical treatment were even more poignant. Piers began his account in the most humble manner, confessing "how utterly futile must have been all my attempts at medical treatment on the upper deck" of the Africans he was entrusted to care for and cure.[103] Even after these fifty healthy Africans were removed from the *Progresso,* conditions were appalling and the number of men in charge of treating the Africans too small, even though they had kept some of the slavers to help them in this task. Soon, Piers commented, sickness "made its appearance amongst our own men, reducing them to only two or three in each watch. . . . Filth was unavoidable . . . and the stench in every part of the vessel was almost intolerable."[104]

In addition to the havoc caused by the various diseases among the Africans and their own men, the passage to the Cape of Good Hope, where the vessel was being taken, was beleaguered by bad weather, including strong gales that flattened the tents erected on deck to care for the women and children, and a drop in temperature that forced many of the Africans to seek refuge in the already overcrowded hold. A journey that should have taken fifteen days turned into a fifty days' odyssey, and every day new cases of dysentery, ulcers, and craw craw were discovered and treated. By the time the *Progresso* made it into Simon's Bay, virtually everyone on board was suffering from some form of ailment, a circumstance that Piers blamed on the deficient diet he was able to offer during the passage.[105]

Overcrowding—found on board most of the slave vessels seized by anti-slave trade patrols after 1820—was in itself a major reason for the spread of disease among Africans and crews. Just as Kittle and Piers were forced to transfer fifty children from the *Progresso* to the *Cleopatra,* the surgeon of HMS

Hydra had no option but to do something similar with "78 little boys and four sick persons" who were lying on the slave deck of the Spanish felucca *Pepito,* captured in March 1845 off Quitta.[106] In other cases, as in those of the Portuguese schooners *Maria da Gloria* and *Arrogante,* entire groups of Africans had to be disembarked at the nearest appropriate location in order to save as many lives as possible.[107]

Even in those cases in which disease was not widespread among the Africans, providing them with a suitable diet was crucial for their successful treatment and recovery. In some cases, cooks from captured slave vessels were retained, as they were regularly able to inform prize officers about the condition of the Africans on board, particularly with regard to their most appropriate diet, which was considered to be "a means of prevention and a cure . . . of much more importance than medicine."[108] For example, in the case of a dhow captured off Mozambique in 1845 by HMS *Mutine,* some of the Portuguese sailors were kept, as they "volunteered to cook and superintend" the Africans they had been carrying before until the vessel arrived at Simon's Bay in the Cape of Good Hope. To the surgeon in charge, T. T. Beveridge, the most pressing need in this case was to provide the Africans with a better "diet and regime," as they had been found emaciated and weakened when the ship was seized.[109] In a similar case, J. J. Donford, prize officer on the schooner *Uncas,* also in 1845, later remarked that he had decided to keep the slavers' cook, who "exerted himself to the utmost, not only in his own department, but in arranging everything connected with the slaves and in keeping them in order."[110]

Captain Wyvill and surgeons Kittle and Piers did something analogous upon capturing and boarding the *Progresso* in 1843. Reverend Pascoe Grenfell Hill, who left a written account of his time aboard HMS *Cleopatra* and the *Progresso,* recalled that some of the Spanish slave traders had been kept to help with the cleaning of the ship, and that they had advised the medical officers of the *Cleopatra* on the most effective ways to use some of the medicines they had on board, including "Macela" (chamomile), "Raiz de Althea" (marsh mallow root), and "Gomma Arabica" (gum Arabic). Hill reported that Antonio, one of the sailors, had explained to him that "the bitter of a strong camomile decoction kills the worms in the stomach, and the mixture of the marsh-mallow and the gum Arabic soothes and strengthens the bowels."[111]

Following the recommendations of the time, prize officers and health practitioners also endeavored to clean and fumigate vessels as soon as it was possible to do so. By all accounts, those vessels affected by epidemic dysentery, like the *Progresso,* presented an additional sanitation problem, as the repeated human discharges contributed to the continuous spread of the disease. Assistant Surgeon Henry Piers stated that "Chloride of lime, hot vinegar and gunpowder, were employed as disinfectants," though he added with regret that "their good effect, if any, could have only been very partial and brief."[112] As we have seen, Alexander Bryson, in his 1847 *Report on the Climate and Principal Diseases of the African Station,* stressed the importance of disinfestation and fumigation of slave ships as soon as they had been seized. Bryson suggested that the use of vinegar and the chloride of lime, the two main means of disinfestation used by Kittle and Piers in the *Progresso,* were inefficacious. Instead he recommended charcoal fires, and if possible a thorough cleaning with chloride of zinc, which was capable of "destroying effluvia arising from animal or vegetable substances in a state of decay."[113]

Once the prize officers in charge of captured ships had established basic hygienic and dietary measures to contain the spread of disease, medical officers were able to focus all of their attention on the best ways of treating the ailments found in each vessel. One of the first actions taken by health practitioners tasked with the attention and care of African slaves and slave-trade ship crews was to inspect the ships for medical supplies and to gather as much information as possible from the health practitioners who had previously been in charge of the slaves.

When vessels had been seized under suspicion of being equipped for the slave trade, the size and contents of medicine chests often determined their fate. For example, in the case of the barque *Bella Angela,* captured by HMS *Dolphin* in the first week of May 1844 and taken to the Cape of Good Hope, prize officer Lieutenant William O'Bryen Hoare subsequently declared that his crew had found "an unusually large medicine chest, which on being examined by the [*Dolphin's*] medical officer" was considered "to contain a much larger quantity of medicine than can possibly required for her pretended voyage, particularly some kinds of medicines generally used in slave vessels."[114] The cases of the *Carolina* and the *Esperanza,* both taken to Sierra Leone only months later, in February and March 1845, respectively, were also decided, to a considerable extent, by the size and contents of their respective medicine chests.[115] Likewise, in 1852, Henry Louey, assistant surgeon on HMS *Vestal,* declared that on board the Spanish schooner *Venus* he had found "a very large medicine-chest, completely fitted and furnished with medicine and surgical instruments, sufficient for a long voyage for a great number of persons. There are also bags of sarsaparilla, which are not at all likely to be required in a coasting vessel."[116] Each of these cases, and the many more recorded by Mixed Commission and Vice-Admiralty courts during the period, attest to the importance given by anti–slave trade patrols to medical supplies found aboard slave trade ships.

It is also plausible to suggest that anti–slave trade patrol medical officers and crews often discussed a wide variety of issues with their slave-trading counterparts. One such exchange was described by Reverend Hill in the mid-1840s, when he noted that the assistant surgeon of HMS *Cleopatra,* Henry Piers, had been unable to restore the health of the Africans found on the *Progresso.* Hill, however, also remarked that there was much to learn from the experience and guidance of the "the slave-dealers, in their selection and application of large stores of medicines found on board the vessel."[117] Many of the medicines found were indeed used by Piers during the passage to the Cape of Good Hope. Among those were the chamomile, castor oil, marsh mallow root, sulfate of quinine, gum Arabic, and a range of purgatives, emollients, and pectorals.[118]

Aboard seized slave ships Africans were subjected to exacting treatments. These could take place below or above deck, and until the ship finally reached port, they were mostly of a palliative character. Dysentery, smallpox, craw craw, various types of fevers, and ophthalmia continued to be the main diseases on board slave trade ships after they had been seized. Treatment of these diseases by anti–slave trade patrol surgeons followed an identical methodology as that used by other health practitioners at sea during the period. Dysentery was broadly treated by a change of diet, reinforced by improved hygiene. Other remedies used included castor oil, ipecacuanha root, and the always-present mercury, often combined with opium.[119]

The only known medication at the time against smallpox was immunization. Anti–slave trade patrol surgeons were limited, just as were their slave-trading counterparts, to the use of various ointments to relieve those affected; they used the same unguents for other skin problems, such as craw craw, measles, and some skin ulcers, including leishmaniasis. Meanwhile, ophthalmia was treated for most of the period with a combination of copper sulfate and silver nitrate—the most effective by all accounts—as well as powdered acetate of lead and sulfate of alumina.

Even in those rare cases where those aboard captured slave vessels were found to be generally healthy, prize officers and anti–slave trade patrol health practitioners were obliged to improve the conditions on board so that whatever little disease they had inherited could be eradicated. The barque *Orion,* for example, was seized with 888 Africans off the coast of West Central Africa in 1859 by HMS *Pluto.* Even though the Africans were suffering less from disease than from prevailing emaciation and widespread debility among them as a result of "a long journey and little food," still eight of them had died in the passage by the time the ship was captured.[120] Alfred S. Pratt, the surgeon in charge of surveying the human cargo and establishing the necessary measures to improve their living conditions, commented that he believed that "rest and a regular diet" would minimize further deaths.[121] Years before, in the case of another vessel coincidentally also called *Orion,* and taken before the Court of Mixed Commission at Rio de Janeiro, the prize officer and surgeon in charge provided every sick African found on board with a blanket, and endeavored to ameliorate their diet by giving them generous rations of oranges, jerked beef, farinha, and other foods.[122] Providing the Africans—and the crews— with a suitable diet, rest, cleanliness, and an appropriate medical attention was, then, the most important and immediate action to be taken by prize officers and health practitioners when taking over slave ships.

In February 1845 Jérôme Félix de Monléon, who had recently been posted to the French West African anti–slave trade squadron as the commander of the brig *La Zèbre,* came upon a slave ship for the first time. Confronted with the reality of a small schooner carrying 420 slaves "pressed likes bales" in a narrow space and "suffering from smallpox," he was perplexed by the horrors before his eyes. Recalling the moment days later, de Monléon wrote in a letter to the Baron de Mackau, "It was the first time I attended such a spectacle, and I cannot tell Your Excellency the impression of pain, disgust, and horror that it had upon me."[123] De Monléon's account of his encounter with a slaver contained most of the concerns raised by anti–slave trade patrol captains and crews who left accounts of their close interactions with slave vessels throughout the Atlantic and Indian worlds after 1820. Overcrowding, emaciation, disease, and other horrors were integral components of their interactions with most of the vessels they seized during this period. In the same letter to the Baron de Mackau, De Monléon also described some of the other main activities expected from an anti–slave trade squadron vessel: patrolling vast areas, surveying the African coast, and confronting the violence associated with armed encounters against slave dealers, both at sea and on land.[124]

Fighting inclement weather, resistant slave dealers, and deadly diseases were just some of the day-to-day hazards that beset anti–slave trade personnel, including health practitioners. As they attempted to bring abolitionist ideas and principles into practice, they were also forced to contend with—and were often complicit in—early imperialist efforts linked to exploration and trade enterprises such as those undertaken on the Niger River, which often resulted in new conflicts and proto-colonial incidents, such as those occurred on the Nuñez River and in Gabon, and that contributed to the growth of forced labor in Africa.

FOUR

"Such an Asylum of Wretchedness"

Anti–Slave Trade Reception Centers, Hospitals, and Cemeteries

One of the party . . . proposed the following toast, which I give verbatim:—
The most usefullest men as is in the colony, I means, the doctors!
—Peter Leonard, *Records of a Voyage to the Western Coast of Africa*

IT WAS DECEMBER 1840, and British practitioner George McHenry
was about to spend his first night as the surgeon of the newly created liberated Africans establishment on the remote Atlantic island of Saint Helena.[1]
The depot, a result of the implementation of new aggressive abolitionist
policies in the Atlantic by the British, had been placed not far from Saint
Helena's capital Jamestown, in Lemon Valley, a venue that was considered
at the time to be the best option for receiving recaptured Africans due to its
geographical position, and to its easy access to both the sea and a stream of
fresh water.[2]

McHenry's first day and night there were not, however, what he had
imagined they would be.[3] Narrating his experiences for a wider public a few
years later in the pages of the *Simmonds' Colonial Magazine and Foreign
Miscellany*, he described what he saw in the makeshift camp where some of
the first Africans landed on the island had been laid down, as "scenes of
misery each succeeding in rivalling the preceding one in some new feature
of hideousness."[4] When the night approached, McHenry made his way to
the captured vessel *Andorinha*, which had been towed to Lemon Valley

only a few days before to serve as a temporary floating ward for those with dysentery and smallpox; there he was faced with more suffering and despair.[5] The first night on the ship left a lasting impression on him. He complained about the absence of a supreme being and reasoned that even God himself would have chosen to stay away from what he called "such an asylum of wretchedness."[6]

McHenry was not able to sleep at all that first night: "Separated from the sick by only a thin partition of deal boards, the groans of the afflicted and shrieks of the dying" did not allow him to do so.[7] Over the next days, weeks, and months, the conditions on Lemon Valley and on the vessels used as provisional hospital wards steadily improved, but only after McHenry himself complained repeatedly to the authorities, emphasizing the need to spend more on this humanitarian project, and to make it a priority among the many issues the island's governor had to contend with.[8] As a matter of fact, he came to describe Lemon Valley with such biblical epithets as the "valley of the shadow of death," a "real Golgotha," and a "place of skulls," when referring to the omnipresence of disease and death among those who inhabited it.[9]

McHenry's disturbing description and narrative of the fate of the Africans processed by the Vice-Admiralty Court of Saint Helena mirrored those offered by other officers and witnesses who left accounts of these establishments across the Atlantic. Wherever Africans were landed, from the Cape of Good Hope to Havana, and from Freetown to Rio de Janeiro, they did so, in the vast majority of the cases, in dreadful conditions, often emaciated and ridden by disease. Tending to their needs, and especially treating their ailments, constituted the work of those engaged in bringing the transatlantic slave trade to an end. On many occasions, these same officers had to treat the slave vessel crews that had been detained, as well as the crews of the cruisers who had brought them to port, as they were just as susceptible to contracting the diseases they had come into contact with whether engaging in the slave trade or its suppression.

In most cases reception centers for liberated Africans were intrinsically linked to Mixed Commission and Vice-Admiralty courts.[10] Whereas the work of these courts was vital in bringing the slave trade to an end and in expanding the British overseas influence and authority, day to day court officers and employees had to interact directly with people who were often plagued by dangerous diseases. To treat them, they created medical facilities, which were always separated from the nearest urban populations by land or water, or both. In Saint Helena, African slaves and slave trade crews were first located in Lemon Valley in 1840, only to be moved to Rupert's Valley, on the other side of the capital, Jamestown, in 1841.[11]

In Sierra Leone, they were sent to the interior of the colony, first to a mountain hospital at the village of Leicester in 1820, and subsequently to Kissy, a short ride from Freetown to the east, where more suitable and resourceful medical installations were built beginning in 1827.[12] In Rio de Janeiro they were regularly kept on the vessels they had arrived or were sent to the infamous Casa de Correção. Later a series of ships that doubled as quarantine and hospital facilities, most notably HMS *Crescent* between 1839 and 1851, were used to host them, until they could be either sent overseas or disembarked in Brazil.[13] A similar system prevailed in Havana, where the detainees were either kept aboard the slave vessels or sent to barracoons outside the perimeter of the city, at least until HMS *Romney* was brought into the harbor in 1837.[14] In other Atlantic ports similar procedures were followed, with medical practitioners always involved to a certain degree in the decision-making process. All in all, these installations became essential not only as weapons in the struggle against the transatlantic slave trade but also as tools in the battle against the deadly diseases associated with it.[15]

Mixed Commission and Vice-Admiralty Courts

The task assigned to the courts of Mixed Commission and Vice-Admiralty during this period was an endeavor comparable in scope to patrolling the Atlantic. These "important but neglected" courts, to use Leslie Bethell's words, were the centerpiece of British abolitionist efforts across the Atlantic and beyond, into the Indian Ocean.[16] Together with the Royal Navy they became the embodiment of how British abolitionism and colonial expansionism were put in practice, and their work often determined whether abolitionist efforts were considered to be worth of continuous funding and support.[17]

After the Napoleonic Wars were over, Britain had the opportunity to exert influence over other European powers that had been affected by the military conflagration. Already at the Congress of Vienna, in 1815, sustained efforts had been made to enact a commitment from all European nations to abolish the slave trade. Although these efforts produced only a joint declaration, lacking the force of a legal document, it was clear that Britain was willing to leverage its superior military and naval power to lead a continent-wide resolution against the slave trade.[18]

Bilateral treaties were signed first with Portugal and Spain in 1817, and with the Netherlands in 1818. Other treaties followed: with Brazil in 1826, France in 1831, and most of the newly formed Latin American republics in the 1820s and 1830s. Only the United States refused to commit to any bilateral agreement with Britain that would effectively allow the British Navy to stop and search any vessel from any signatory country suspected of being involved in the transatlantic slave trade.[19] Bilateral treaties were also imposed on numerous African rulers, allowing for the British to use gunboat diplomacy whenever the African signatories violated their terms. The most notorious action of this kind taken was the bombardment and occupation of Lagos in 1851, which soon led to the establishment of a British protectorate, and eventually to its annexation in 1861.[20]

Many of the Mixed Commission courts did little or no work, as ships from the nations involved were seldom or never taken to them. Some Latin American countries did not even host courts in their own territories, relinquishing that right to the British, who habitually hosted their branches of most courts at Sierra Leone. The appearances of Latin American slave vessels—Brazilian ones excepted—before the Mixed Commission Court in Freetown were rare events, as only the *Izabel* in 1851 and the *Constancia* in 1861 were ever processed there.[21]

As a result of the breakdown of negotiations between Britain and Portugal in the late 1830s, the Palmerston Act of 1839 allowed Royal Navy vessels to intercept and search Portuguese ships and flagless ships suspected of participating in the slave trade. These vessels were taken to Vice-Admiralty courts, which were consequently charged with this new responsibility. The

1839 act supplemented the equipment clause signed with Spain as part of the new bilateral treaty of 1835, which also gave the British the right to stop and search any Spanish vessel deemed to be equipped for the slave trade, and to adjudicate cases against its owners.[22]

Unlike Vice-Admiralty courts, where the British single-handedly judged and adjudicated cases against slave traders, Mixed Commission courts, especially those that at least for a time functioned with some degree of efficiency, were formed by two sets of officers representing the British and the cosignatory nations of each treaty.[23] The various courts at Freetown—Anglo-Portuguese, Anglo-Spanish, Anglo-Brazilian, Anglo-Dutch—were by far the busiest. The courts established at Havana and Rio de Janeiro were the only others that held significant numbers of hearings beginning in the early 1820s.[24] Adjudicating against slave ships captured by anti-slave trade patrols, and "disposing" of the Africans found on board as legal prizes, made up the work of the Mixed Commission, and later of the Vice-Admiralty courts.

Coping with limited resources and a wide array of impediments that ranged from disruptive local authorities to deadly epidemics, Mixed Commission courts continued to function until they were gradually disbanded and replaced by Vice-Admiralty courts from the 1840s onward. Disease and death were ever-present problems for court officers, irrespective of their Atlantic locations. Alongside judges, clerks, registrars, and interpreters, Mixed Commission and Vice-Admiralty courts always counted at least one health practitioner among their ranks. Receiving, treating, revitalizing, and relocating severely disease-stricken men, women, and children were central to the success of the courts' operations.

Such relocations often involved a sort of second Middle Passage toward the British West Indies, where recaptured human cargoes were subjected to a new sort of indentured labor system disguised as benevolent apprenticeship. In other cases, many of the men were recruited from Freetown's Liberated Africans Yard, even before they had completely recovered, in order to swell the ranks of the British West India Regiment.[25]

But dealing with disease and death was not an abstract concept to those involved with the courts. In Sierra Leone alone, several officers belonging to both the courts of Mixed Commission and Vice-Admiralty died during the period, and there is little doubt that virtually every single person working there suffered from the notorious fevers of the African coast, and from other potentially lethal diseases. In addition to the frightening epidemics of yellow fever that attacked Sierra Leone in 1823, 1829–30, 1837, and 1847, seasonal fevers, usually malaria and typhoid, were frequent.

Indeed, most of the first officers sent to Freetown from Spain, Portugal, the Netherlands, and Britain either died or fled in panic, fearing for their lives. Portuguese commissioners João Jacomo de Altavilla and Joaquim Cesar de la Figanière were forced to leave Sierra Leone almost as soon as they arrived, in order to "escape from an almost certain death," as they were both attacked by the fevers of the country.[26] Altavilla fell ill barely forty-eight hours after landing, and before abandoning his post, he grumbled profusely about the "abominable climates of the Sierra Leone peninsula."[27] Spanish commissioners José Camps and Francisco Lefer Robaud were also attacked by fevers soon after their arrival. In their letters to Madrid they complained that the resulting weaknesses hindered their capacity to carry out their work at the Anglo-Spanish Mixed Commission Court. Lefer Robaud, in particular, lamented having been attacked by the fever four times since his arrival, although he also rejoiced at being alive, as he observed that sixty-eight Europeans had died since he had landed in Freetown.[28] Even British commissioner Edward Gregory, who in late 1824 had boasted of having been favored by "some kind of providence" that had kept him relatively healthy since his arrival five years earlier, eventually fell ill and died soon after predicting that such a long residence in Freetown was likely to prove fatal.[29]

Other African spots where courts were set up, such as Cape Verde, Luanda, and the Cape of Good Hope Colony, also were perilous. On the American side, while Rio de Janeiro was until the late 1840s presumed to be the healthiest of all locations, Havana was never accorded such a reputation.[30] The Cuban capital was considered to be an insalubrious place, and was described as such by Robert Jameson, the first Mixed Commission court judge to land there, in 1820. Jameson decried the city's predisposition for "the propagation and retention of disease."[31] Around the time Jameson wrote this comment, Havana had suffered frequent yellow fever outbreaks, and the disease was a constant threat to the health and lives of those who lived or stopped in the city, as French visitor Mr. Deliège in 1819 commented upon his return to Paris:

> I have just arrived back from Havana, which I had to leave at once because of Vomito Negro before I had time to complete the personal businesses that took me there; this terrible plague has, between the 1st April and 15th May, wiped out 76 French people, excluding foreigners.[32]

Yellow fever was hardly the only dangerous disease affecting Havana in the first half of the nineteenth century, as smallpox, typhus, and two epidemics of cholera attacked the city throughout the period. Only a few years after Jameson and Deliège wrote about the ravages of yellow fever in the Cuban capital, South Carolinian visitor Abiel Abbot recorded his observations about another common disease, dengue fever, which he considered to be the "most singular disease endemic in the place."[33] Abbot went on to remark that this was "a disease chiefly of the bones," which crippled "its subjects' hands and feet."[34]

Just as was the case with slave ports and factories, and vessels of all kinds, the Atlantic spots chosen as battlegrounds for the struggle against the human traffic in the Atlantic were at the heart of contact zones ridden with disease and subjected to strict sanitation measures implemented in the vain hope of containing disease. Mixed Commission and Vice-Admiralty courts acted as transdimensional bridges between the legal and illegal realms that existed across the Atlantic world. The paperwork they left behind constitutes one of the most remarkable bodies of information about how the slave trade was carried out and fought against after 1820. This paperwork also illustrates how disease was fought by a wide array of practitioners and other ordinary people throughout the Atlantic and how medical knowledge was used by a number of non-African states and nations to stake territorial claims to several parts of Africa.

Anti–Slave Trade Reception Centers

Shortly after their arrival in ports like Freetown, Rio de Janeiro, Havana, Jamestown, Luanda, or the Cape Colony, all seized slave trade vessels were to undergo a medical inspection, usually conducted by a medical officer attached to one of the Mixed Commission or Vice-Admiralty courts. These medical officers would normally go on board the ships, accompanied by African interpreters and, on occasion, by court officers, to determine the health of those on board, including crews and slaves, and to establish the right course of action to follow, depending on whether the ship and its passengers posed a threat to the local population of the port.[35]

Those Africans who were deemed to be fit and well were normally landed and taken to specific abodes where they could recover their lost strength. In Sierra Leone, where the British were in control of all proceedings, the preferred place to disembark them was the Liberated Africans Yard—also known as King's Yard or Queen's Yard, depending on the year and the reigning monarch. The yard was purposely sited near the water, to the west of the rest of the city, in the hope that such a leeward location would prevent dispersal of any diseases they might have brought with them.[36] Although the space given to pen the newly arrived Africans was supposed to be large enough as to provide them with opportunities to exercise and recover, in the eyes of a contemporary visitor the place was nothing short of "a large species of prison . . . encompassed by high walls, and secured by well-guarded gates."[37]

In spite of the attempts made by the local authorities to create a safe environment based on the location of the yard and the attentions given to the recently landed Africans, the site was still a source of anxiety to the residents of Freetown. In 1829, Thomas Cole, superintendent of liberated Africans, wrote to Acting Governor Henry Ricketts reporting that the closest neighbors had been "considerably alarmed," and had attributed the cause of the fevers raging at the time in the colony to the "distemper imported by those people."[38] As we have seen, the yard also became a favorite haunt for the officers of the West India Regiment looking to add new recruits to their ranks. In 1827, Dixon Denham, who was the predecessor of

Cole as superintendent of liberated Africans, continued to encourage this policy in his official correspondence with Colonel Hugh Lumley, suggesting that "some of the men would be desirable recruits" for his corps.[39] As soon as authorities saw fit, the recaptured Africans who were considered to be in good health would be then transferred to one of the villages in the Freetown's hinterland.[40]

In Saint Helena, where the British were also in charge of receiving the Africans freed from apprehended slave vessels after the Palmerston Act came into effect in 1840, colonial officers were forced to improvise. As we have seen, they created facilities first in Lemon Valley to the west, then in Rupert's Valley, to the east of the capital, Jamestown. The haste with which these installations were assembled, and the sudden influx of large numbers of recaptured Africans, led to several crises, and to the implementation of inadequate measures to separate the healthy from the sick. Crowded conditions were often reported from the moment Lemon Valley facilities were set up in 1840, which led John Young, collector of customs at Jamestown, to ask Governor George Middlemore "that separate accommodations at Lemon Valley be provided whereby the healthy shall be removed from the diseased."[41] Over the years, and in spite of the efforts of colonial officers and health practitioners like doctors George McHenry, Christopher Vowell, James Rawlins, Henry Solomon, and others, conditions improved only partially.[42]

In Rio de Janeiro, where first the Portuguese and then the Brazilian authorities determined to a larger extent the fate of the recaptured Africans, those who were deemed to be healthy enough to be landed were often sent to either the Casa de Correção or the Depósito Geral da Cidade, or in some cases were placed with private citizens.[43] The situation in Havana, the other major slave-trading port with a Mixed Commission court, was similar. There, after careful examination and for most of the period, healthy slaves were placed in the Depósito de Cimarrones, located in the El Cerro neighborhood, or in other barracoons, usually owned and guarded by private citizens.[44] In both cases, British officers attached to the courts protested repeatedly about the poor conditions of the establishments offered by their hosts to newly arrived Africans, as well as to the Royal Navy and slave vessels' crews.[45]

Whereas those Africans who were considered to be healthy enough were landed at major cities and placed in urban quarters until their fate could be decided, those who were found to be sickly received an altogether different treatment, which included seclusion in isolated quarantine lazarettos and vessels, or relocation to other medical facilities like hospitals, including hospital vessels. In Sierra Leone, quarantine ships were used early on to separate sickly Africans and crews from the rest of the population. A common practice was to leave those who were considered to be suffering from infectious diseases on board the same vessels they had arrived in, while immediately removing those considered to be healthy. In this way, slave vessels often doubled as quarantine ships.

In a letter sent to Foreign Secretary George Canning in October 1826, Commissioner Daniel Hamilton described the measures taken upon the arrival of the brig *Perpetuo Defensor*. The ship had reached Sierra Leone carrying a large number of Africans suffering from diarrhea, dysentery, and smallpox. After informing Canning about the removal of the healthy from the vessel, Hamilton explained that the rest were to be placed under quarantine on the same ship.[46] In order to avoid mishaps, the colonial surgeon, at the time Robert Boyle, recommended to Colonial Secretary Joseph Reffell that he order the prize officer to keep a yellow flag constantly hoisted, to avoid communications between the ship and the shore, to warn any boats seen approaching the vessel away from the risk they were taking, and to fire a gun in the event of requiring anything, so that the quarantine boat could be sent to assist.[47]

In addition to the quarantine ships, in February 1827 a lazaretto or quarantine facility was built at Kissy, a few miles east of Freetown, where the most severe cases of disease could be contained. This new lazaretto was situated by the waterside at a place where slave vessels could dock without much trouble, and in close proximity to the new Kissy hospital for the reception of liberated Africans.[48] In the early 1830s, Peter Leonard described the site as nothing more than "a few huts . . . surrounded by a wall."[49] Not long after, Harrison Rankin reported that sickly slaves were now being separated from those who were healthy, and being "conveyed to the lazaretto out of the town."[50] A few years later, in the mid-1840s, Robert Clarke referred to the lazaretto as the "lower hospital," contrasting it to the "upper hospital," where the other liberated Africans were accommodated.[51] According to Clarke, the six-foot wall that surrounded the site was already a stone structure by the time he arrived there. He also commented that annexed to it there was a "grass-house, for the reception of the cases where the cure is tedious."[52]

While the establishment of quarantine installations in Sierra Leone was relatively well planned and undertaken in stages, the situation in Saint Helena bordered on desperate at times. There, colonial officers and medical practitioners were under heavy pressure to provide basic quarantine facilities from the moment when sickly Africans began to arrive in 1840. While the Medical Board initially recommended using Egg Island, an inhospitable rock situated to the southwest of Jamestown, as the most desirable site to receive those affected with the most serious cases of infectious diseases, the proposal was soon discarded, as the place did not fulfill the most basic requirements to administer the medical provision of those who would be placed there.[53] After some discussion, it was agreed that Lemon Valley, a site that had traditionally been "the default location for the quarantine of sick arrivals to the island," be used to receive those who arrived suffering of infectious maladies.[54] In addition to Lemon Valley, over the years a number of vessels also served as quarantine ships. In fact, almost simultaneously with the choice of Lemon Valley as a reception and quarantine center, two slave vessels, the *Andorinha* and the *Julia,* were designated to function as quarantine stations as well.[55]

Over the years Rupert's Valley became the main reception center for the newly arrived recaptured Africans, often combining quarantine facilities with a hospital and a depot. Throughout the 1840s, however, those in charge of caring for new arrivals were relentless in their complaints. McHenry, who was in charge of Lemon Valley, repeatedly called the attention of the authorities to the poor sanitation and the lax quarantine measures there. In April 1842 he lamented that the installations under his control counted "twenty eight different dwellings, two ships, eighteenth tents, and eight different houses or huts, altogether extended over a space of about half a mile in length."[56] As a result, he asserted, men, women, and children had found themselves sleeping in the open, ungoverned by the quarantine measures he had put in place. A year later, he wrote a direct letter to the secretary for the colonies, the Earl of Derby, describing his predicament, which included taking care of 70 patients a day as an average, and some days as many as 320, who had been "distributed on board of two, three, four, and five vessels, besides the shore."[57]

Over the years, Lemon Valley was slowly but steadily abandoned in favor of Rupert's Valley, where overall conditions were significantly better for the reception of both healthy and sickly Africans.[58] Prize vessels continued to be used as quarantine stations for years to come. In early 1848 the *Gentil Africano* was captured by HMS *Styx* and taken to Saint Helena, where it was condemned as being equipped for the slave trade.[59] The ship was soon destined to serve as a quarantine station and as a hospital in a case of emergency.[60] Days later it underwent an extensive transformation, having all decks relaid, with the aim of offering better conditions for receiving new groups of recaptured Africans.[61] In subsequent years quarantine provision continued to be administered through permanent buildings and temporary tents in Rupert's Valley, as well as quarantine vessels, which continued to be the subject of debate among colonial authorities and the functionaries involved with medical provision.[62]

In Rio de Janeiro and Havana, where the British largely had to abide by local laws, organizing quarantines was often a subject for negotiation with the Portuguese, Brazilian, and Spanish authorities. In Rio de Janeiro, those recaptured Africans who arrived suffering from infectious diseases were regularly kept on board the ships they had arrived in, while those who were deemed healthy were landed and taken to the Casa de Correção, the Depósito Geral, or some other detention site.[63] Beginning in the mid-1830s, a decommissioned Portuguese galley anchored inside Guanabara Bay, the *Nova Piedade,* began to function simultaneously as a quarantine station and hospital ship for the recaptured Africans and as a prison for the crews of the slave vessels captured.[64] By the end of the 1830s the *Nova Piedade,* now a crumbling hulk, was considered to be "very ill adapted," for the purpose that was then serving, and a new vessel, HMS *Crescent,* was sent from Britain to replace it.[65]

The *Crescent* soon became indispensable for the reception and treatment of recaptured Africans, while also serving, as the *Nova Piedade* had done before, as a prison for the slave vessels' crews. While British Consul

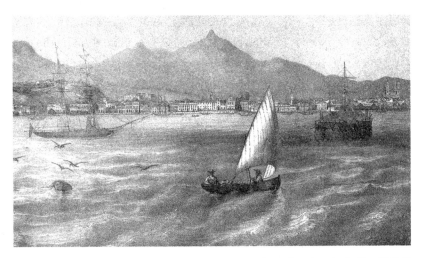

Fig. 15. View of Rio de Janeiro and Guanabara harbor, showing the hulk of HMS *Crescent* on the right. NMM: SOG; RRK; E; 5; Box 0998.

Ouseley praised the effectiveness of the *Crescent* a short time after its arrival, some of the slave-trade sailors who had been imprisoned in its lower decks complained profusely about the poor hygienic conditions on board. Ouseley, who had previously insisted on using the *Crescent* for a variety of purposes, was quick to point out to Viscount Palmerston in September 1840 that since its arrival at Rio de Janeiro the "maladies peculiar to the negroes [had] disappeared or nearly so" once they had been transferred to the ship.[66] On the other hand, only a few months later, in February 1841, the brother of João Baptista Boisson, who had been retained on the *Crescent* after being found aboard the *Asseisseira,* supposedly as a passenger, requested permission to disembark his brother so that he could receive appropriate treatment for his ailments and escape the "fetid" atmosphere of the *Crescent* created by the Africans, which, in his opinion, was "augmenting his anguish."[67] Throughout the 1840s and almost until the end of the transatlantic slave trade to Brazil, the *Crescent* continued to provide a political and epidemiological challenge for Brazilian authorities.[68]

In Havana during this period the situation was much different, as the Spanish colonial authorities exerted a much greater influence in determining the most appropriate sites for quarantined Africans and crews. Unlike Rio de Janeiro, Havana had long developed methods of fending off dangerous diseases. After the Mixed Commission Court began receiving vessels full of sick African slaves, Cuban authorities took the initiative, designating specific places outside the limits of the city, where those infected could recover without transmitting their diseases to the rest of the population. Although in some cases, ailing Africans were kept on board the same ships they had come in, or were sent to the depot of El Príncipe, near the country house of the captain generals, the preferred quarantine destination for most of the period was a series of barracks, or barracones, located between the castle of La Punta and the Vedado area, to the west of the city and by the sea.[69] These notoriously unhealthy barracoons had been used to receive enslaved Africans since the late eighteenth or early nineteenth century. When José Fernández de Madrid visited them in 1817, just weeks after Spain committed to abolishing the slave trade, he recalled seeing "a number of dying blacks naked and spread out on wooden planks, many of them reduced to skin and bones, and inhaling an intolerable stench."[70] A continuous flow of sick Africans found their way to these receptacles. For example, in July 1829 the smallpox-afflicted Africans who arrived in the ship *Midas* were immediately sent by Governor Francisco Dionisio Vives to the Vedado barracks, so that Havana could be kept "safe from the ravages that might be occasioned by a disease so contagious."[71] Even after the arrival of HMS *Romney* in Havana in 1837, those Africans who had entered the harbor laboring under infectious diseases continued to be sent to these barracks outside the city perimeter, as the *Romney* apparently was not equipped to deal appropriately with cases that required strict quarantines.[72]

In other Atlantic destinations, quarantines were also dutifully kept, often on board infected vessels or on land. For example, in Fernando Po, quarantined vessels and people were sent to Point Adelaide, near Port Clarence, until they were considered to be risk-free.[73] In New York, a quarantine ground was firmly established by the mid-1840s at Long Island, and at the Cape of Good Hope, where a lazaretto was never properly established, quarantines were usually undertaken in Simon's Bay, at "two batteries, close to the beach."[74]

A final and fundamental type of medical facility, hospitals, whenever they were established, were central for the appropriate functioning of Mixed Commission and Vice-Admiralty courts. Like lazarettos, hospitals could be founded in convenient locations, relatively isolated from large populations, or, alternatively, could be established on ships, occasionally on some of those captured with enslaved Africans. In truth, hospitals and lazarettos, just like hospital ships and "floating lazarettos," did, at times, fulfill similar duties all over the Atlantic. In Sierra Leone, between 1820 and 1827, British authorities operated a hospital for liberated Africans in some former school buildings that had been abandoned by missionaries at the mountain village of Leicester. Although in principle, the high position of Leicester would have made this an ideal location for this type of facility, in reality both the place and the inappropriateness of the existing buildings came under repeated criticism. Soon after taking charge in 1820, Joseph Reffell had to undertake a program of comprehensive refurbishment to make the buildings fit for their new purpose, and a few months later, in March 1821, he was forced to employ an engineer to carry out further extensive repairs.[75] By 1826, most of health practitioners residing in Sierra Leone were quick to point out the inadequacies of this hospital through a questionnaire sent to them by the Sierra Leone Commission of Enquiry, led by James Rowan and Henry Wellington.[76] William Barry, principal medical officer on the west coast of Africa, considered the buildings "very unfit for [their] purpose, particularly for newly arrived negroes," on account of being placed in a very high location, and always being cold and damp.[77] As a matter of fact, Barry suggested that the hospital be moved to the river village of Kissy. William Ferguson also criticized Leicester hospital for being "at too great an altitude above the level of the sea, and totally inadequate as a building for the reception of the sick."[78] The surgeon to the Forces, Alexander Stewart, gave a similar assessment of the buildings and their location.[79]

Perhaps as a direct result of this set of answers, including Barry's suggestion, the hospital at Leicester was closed for good at the end of January 1827 and moved to Kissy, following the late Governor Sir Neil Campbell's orders.[80] On the first day of February, a new "building was assigned, near the waterside, for the reception of the sick distressed Liberated Africans from the villages and for such newly arrived people from slave vessels."[81]

The new hospital at Kissy was in its origins nothing but a mixture of crumbling houses. When compared to the structures at Leicester, however, those at Kissy seemed to have been much more solid and to have offered a potential for expansion and development that was impossible at Leicester. In September 1829, Thomas Cole described the place as "a stone building" capable of receiving at once more than two hundred people.[82]

Over the next decades, the Kissy hospital came to play an enormously important role in the Atlantic campaign for abolishing the slave trade. Perhaps more than any other medical facility, Kissy hosted large numbers of Africans, which in practice meant that it had to be continuously supplied and developed. The small, limited stone edifices inherited by the hospital in 1827 were soon expanded into a group of buildings, surrounded by a wall, and a burial ground. Colonial practitioners tightly ran the hospital, although from its early days complaints were voiced about corruption and lack of discipline.[83] Patients were inspected daily, admissions and diet books were kept up to date, and medical attention was dispensed by a collection of British practitioners and African employees, many of whom were recruited from the ranks of newly arrived liberated Africans.[84]

From the beginning, keeping the place clean and organized was a central endeavor for all those involved in the running of the hospital. Repairs were constant, and expansion continued for years. When Peter Leonard visited Kissy in the early 1830s, he referred to the hospital as "a range of low buildings," which he considered to be "ill adapted for the purposes of a hospital."[85] Harrison Rankin, who visited the colony in 1834, described the place as a "fever hospital," which was "insulated, and with an enclosure bounded by high walls."[86] The most detailed description of the hospital's evolution over time was given in the 1840s by Robert Clarke, who made references to two well-defined sets of buildings. One was the lower hospital or lazaretto, which was situated by the sea, and the other the upper hospital, situated in a more elevated setting.[87]

The upper hospital was, in Clarke's words, "a quadrangular stone building with semi-circular additions at both ends, plus other minor additions, including a kitchen and quarters for the employees."[88] By this time those in charge of the hospital had been forced to create a new ward for

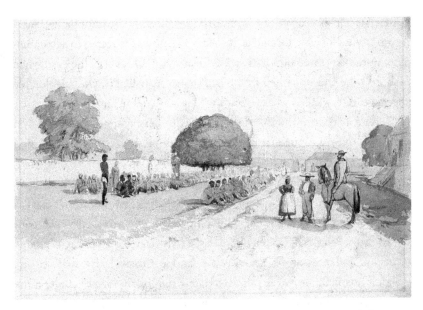

Fig. 16. Landing Africans seized by HMS *Spitfire,* c. 1860. Kissy Hospital. NMM: ZBA2731.

mentally ill patients, some of whom arrived in virtually every vessel. The ward was separated from the rest of the buildings and located "near the women's side of the hospital."[89] The buildings were contained within an area of about two hundred square feet, which was enclosed by a white-washed fourteen-foot-high wall; the compound was supposedly capable of receiving up to five hundred individuals at a time.

Kissy hospital continued to function until the 1860s, when the slave trade in the Atlantic basin was finally brought to an end.[90] A watercolor from September 1859 is the only contemporary graphic image we have of this important site: the artwork depicts a group of liberated Africans out-side the hospital, some sitting and others standing, soon after their seizure aboard the slave ship *J. Harris* and subsequent debarkation at Kissy.

In Saint Helena, where most of the Africans caught on ships bound for the Americas after 1840 in the South Atlantic were taken, another hospital was built with the intention of replacing the makeshift reception centers at Lemon and Rupert's valleys, and the temporary wards created on adjudicated slave vessels, which also served at the same time as off-shore quarantine stations.[91] At times, the hospital, located at Rupert's Valley, was required to accommodate more than three hundred sick Africans at once, as was the case when Bishop Robert Gray visited in the late 1840s. Appalled by the "deplorable spectacle," Gray called what he saw the "master work of Satan."[92]

As it had been the case in Sierra Leone, discussions about the best place to locate the hospital started practically from the moment the first Africans arrived in the colony in 1840. As Lemon Valley proved to be inadequate for the reception and medical attention of those Africans and slave-ship crews suffering from infectious diseases, Rupert's Valley was chosen as the best-suited site to replace it. When the long and narrow valley was converted into a reception center, eleven large tents were erected, each capable of accommodating around 30 people, and a three-ward "single-storey, wooden hospital, measuring approximately 6 m by 60 m," was built at the back of the area where the tents were placed.[93] Twelve additional tents were situated along the wooden building, specifically destined for convalescing Africans. The hospital was enclosed by a low stone wall and could receive up to 140 patients at a time.[94]

Over the next two decades repeated attempts to upgrade the hospital and other facilities at Rupert's Valley led nowhere, as metropolitan authorities in London refused to allow any major investment. In spite of these setbacks, the hospital was annually cleaned and whitewashed, and small repairs were continuously made to maintain the standards necessary to provide the medical service for which it was intended.[95] Rupert's Valley hospital continued to function until the 1860s, at times supported by hospital vessels like the *Volant* or the *Gentil Africano,* and by Jamestown hospital.[96] Just as had been the case in Sierra Leone, before long, as large numbers of Africans landed immediately after suffering the traumatic experience of the Middle Passage, the establishment of a mental ward became necessary. The Sandy Bay Lunatics Asylum was created soon after and continued to operate until the late 1840s or early 1850s at Sandy Bay, on the south side of the island.[97]

As we have seen, at Rio de Janeiro, those Africans suffering from contagious diseases were either kept on board the vessels they had arrived in or sent, almost immediately, to the *Nova Piedade* or the *Crescent,* where they were nurtured until they had recovered enough to continue their journey toward the British West Indies or to be relocated within Brazilian society.[98] Both the *Nova Piedade* and the *Crescent* functioned as quarantine and hospital wards, as well as temporary prisons for slave-ship crews.[99] The limited space provided by these vessels and the fact that they were used for multiple purposes led to more human suffering among newly arrived Africans. In the Mixed Commission court session of January 13, 1837, British officers raised their concerns about the "lack of air, space, cleanliness and treatment" to which Africans were exposed, leading to "more misery and to the mortality that has taken place aboard the detained vessels, so that they were suffering more now than during their [transatlantic] voyages."[100]

Certainly, Rio de Janeiro was not devoid of hospitals or medical practitioners. The Casa da Misericordia was considered to be a modern hospital, situated not far from the Casa de Correção and the Depósito Geral. According to Robert Walsh, who visited the city in the late 1820s, a considerable number of health practitioners lived there at the time, including more than one hundred surgeons, some of them French and British.[101] In Rio de Janeiro authorities had in place a number of questionable health measures, which suggested that when it came to preventing potentially devastating diseases, much emphasis was on offering the illusion of being in control. The Regimento de Saúde or Health Regulations of July 9, 1833, for example, had, according to Jaime Rodrigues, only a minuscule effect.[102] Bills of Health were also frequently found in slave vessels, although as Rodrigues has pointed out, "they always certified as good the conditions of the ports and the ships, freeing them to continue their voyage."[103]

At the time, Havana also was home to a number of hospitals of different sizes and quality, including the Military Hospital, which was considered "one of the finest in the world."[104] The city had been dealing with infectious diseases from the early years of the Spanish colonization, and thus its medical authorities had devised systems, including quarantine and hospital wards, specifically dedicated to controlling contagion when outbreaks occurred or were anticipated.[105]

As the Anglo-Spanish Court of Mixed Commission began its labors in Havana in the early 1820s, sick slaves represented but one of the many problems they had to address on a regular basis. Rather than leaving all medical treatment to the physicians attached to the court and, from 1837 to the *Romney*, Cuban authorities often proactively agreed to land those Africans suffering from infectious diseases, with the clear intention of having total control over their movement and the possible spread of their diseases. For this reason, they relied on the barracoons of El Vedado, and for those who were deemed not to be of the highest risk, other barracoons such as the one under the care of Ramón Morales, located near the country house of the island's governors.[106]

British Mixed Commission officers, as well as British consuls, super-intendents of liberated Africans, and other functionaries, often went happily along with the dispositions of the Spanish authorities regarding treatment of newly arrived Africans with infectious diseases. This surrender of powers to the authorities of Havana on occasion hindered the work of the court, as was the case in 1835, when it was unable to access the ship *Diligencia,* which the port authorities had placed in quarantine, officially out of limits to anyone but their own medical officers.[107] After 1837, however, the *Romney* became the regular destination for newly arrived Africans, who, apart from a few occasions in which the chances of contagion were deemed too high, were habitually sent there regardless of the state of their health.[108]

In other Atlantic locations where recaptured Africans were taken, which lacked the resources of local authorities and courts of Mixed Commission and Vice-Admiralty, they were usually treated in quarantine stations or in general hospitals. In some places, like Fernando Po, site of an attempt to re-settle the Sierra Leone Mixed Commission Court in the late 1820s, a hospital was erected near Fort William in 1827, adapted to receive sick Africans as well as crews and formed by "two small houses, each twenty feet square."[109] The isolated situation of Fort William had been considered ideal by Captain William Owen, "as it was near the extreme point of a small peninsula, on which prevailing winds [blew] transversely."[110] Fernando Po's geographical location had also been instrumental in the attempt to make the Spanish territory the epicenter of British abolitionism in West Africa: not only was it conveniently situated much closer to the Bights, but it was considered to be "the only place upon the whole line of the coast upon which hospitals and other conveniences could be erected, far above the reach of the coast fever."[111] By the mid-1840s, the building had been almost completely abandoned, although according to William Daniell, its isolated location, far from the town and exposed to a "reinvigorating sea breeze," was still its main redeeming feature.[112]

At Cape Colony, where considerable numbers of recaptured Africans began to arrive after 1840, quarantine stations were created whenever necessary, as well as a "sizeable hospital" at Simon's Bay, able to receive all those who arrived suffering from disease during these years.[113] In other British colonial spots such as the Gambia, Ascension Island, and Cape Coast, hospitals of various sizes were also built to deal with the occasional arrival of recaptured Africans or slave vessel and Royal Navy sick crews. These installations were not always up to the most basic standards. The hospital of Ascension, for example, was conveniently situated near the garrison, and frequently serviced the West African squadron as well as a number of slave trade vessels' crews in this period.[114] Ascension was considered at the time as the best place to take the sick and the convalescent for recovery.[115] During these years the Gambia also was the site of a military hospital in Bathurst, though it was often criticized by those who visited it. In the late 1840s Thomas Eyre Poole referred to it as a "miserable apology for a refuge for the invalided sufferer," unequal to offering basic comfort and safety to its patients.[116] Only a few years later, Richard Burton complained of the hospital's location, near a swamp, and considered it the place to be "murderous."[117] At the same time, a hospital on the Gold Coast, within the walls of Cape Coast castle, was mostly dedicated to treat the personnel of the British settlement there and the crews of some slave vessels.[118]

In Luanda, where an Anglo-Portuguese Mixed Commission court functioned from the 1840s onward, the *Hospital da Misericordia* had the duty of treating and caring for all those arriving in the Portuguese colony with infectious diseases, including recaptured Africans.[119] The hospital was situated near the church of Santo Antonio, and was, according to those who described it, in a dilapidated state, considered nothing more than "a point of transition between life and death."[120]

Each of these reception centers had at least one more necessary space: the one dedicated to burying the bodies of those Africans and crew members who died upon arrival. In Sierra Leone, as the hospital was moved to Kissy in 1827, a new cemetery was consecrated on the slopes toward the nearby river. In that place were buried missionaries, medical practitioners, and crews belonging to Royal Navy and slave trading vessels, as well as christened Africans. After visiting the burial ground, an evidently impressed Robert Clarke commented that in this place reposed, side by side, "the ashes of the mixed Ethiopic races, mingling their dust with their slave-dealing oppressors; natives of Portugal, Spain, America, &c."[121] For those Africans who died before being baptized, an unconsecrated ground was designated toward the back of the lower hospital. When he referred to the place, Clarke remarked that the cemetery was not walled—unlike the one in consecrated soil nearby—and that the "Pagan Liberated Africans" buried there were being interred without coffins.[122]

In Saint Helena, the cemetery for recaptured Africans in Rupert's Valley was formed by "two large graveyards dating from 1840 to the early 1860s" to replace the original designated burial ground in Lemon Valley near Chamberlain Cottage, and to eliminate the practice of burying some of those who had died at sea.[123] Due to the lack of space these two burial grounds were placed near the inhabited areas and were often a matter of concern for those in charge of the recaptured Africans, as well as for the colonial authorities in Jamestown. The graveyards at Rupert's Valley were excavated in successive archaeological campaigns between 2008 and 2012 by a team led by archeologist Andrew Pearson. The results of these archaeological works were remarkable. Even though most of the bodies seem to have been buried with urgency in shallow graves that often contained two or three bodies, the human remains recovered at the site have confirmed the presence of certain diseases, like scurvy. More striking, however, was the discovery of apparent bone fractures in more than half of adult male skeletons, almost certainly related to the violence of the Middle Passage.[124]

In other British colonies like the Gambia and Ascension, crews from Royal Navy slave trade vessels and liberated Africans were buried in designated cemeteries, which, like those at Kissy and Rupert's Valley, were not always kept in the best conditions. The burial ground at Bathurst in the Gambia seems to have been just as dilapidated as the hospital was. When J.

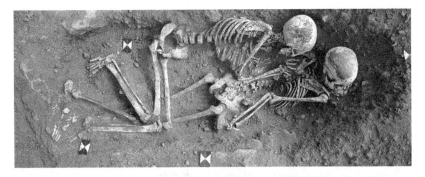

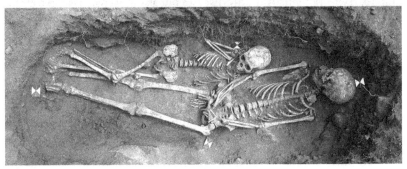

Figs. 17 and 18. Burials at Rupert's Valley. Courtesy of Andrew Pearson.

F. Napier Hewett visited the place in the early 1860s, he mentioned its wrecked state as well as the fact that by all accounts its grounds were "twice the size of the town."[125] Ascension, in spite of its reputation for being a healthier place than any neighboring colony, also had an extensive cemetery where many sailors and officers were buried.

As Pearson has noted, several British vessels suffering from outbreaks of disease sailed to Ascension as the best available destination for arresting the development of these diseases. Among them were HMS *Owen Glendower* and HMS *Bann* in 1823, HMS *Eden* and HMS *Sybille* in 1829, HMS *Black Joke* in 1830, and HMS *Bonetta* in 1838.[126] Crews of vessels detained for being involved in the slave trade or piracy were also sometimes taken there, as was the case for the crew of the *Panda,* in 1833, just before all their members were accused of attacking the American merchant vessel *Mexican* in 1832 and deported to the United States to face trial.[127] The Ascension cemetery, better known as the Bonetta cemetery, was located in "a depression surrounded by a landscape of jagged rock and volcanic ash," and in it were laid to rest the bodies of a large number of officers and crews belonging to the West African squadron who perished there in the spring of 1838.[128]

A similar cemetery was erected on the notoriously unhealthy island of Fernando Po after the British began their ill-fated attempt to take possession of the island and transfer the Sierra Leone courts of Mixed Commission there. Fernando Po not only received many Royal Navy and slave-trade ships carrying potentially deadly diseases but also served as a camp base for the Niger expeditions of the 1830s and 1840s. In the mid-1840s the cemetery, where a number of famous explorers had been buried, including Richard Lander and Bird Allen, was said to be "half-concealed by thickets and dense masses of foliage."[129] The cemetery had been all but abandoned, and a "luxuriant carpet of grass and weeds" covered its grounds.[130]

In Rio de Janeiro, until 1830 recaptured Africans were frequently buried on the grounds of the Cemitério dos Pretos Novos, located on Pedro Ernesto Street, near the quarantine station at Gamboa and the slave market at Valongo. This site has also been excavated in recent years.[131] After the cemetery was closed in 1830, Africans began to be buried in other locations in or around the city, notably in the Cemitério da "Ladeira da Misericórdia."[132]

In Luanda, where an Anglo-Portuguese Mixed Commission was active between 1844 and 1870, recaptured Africans who died after being emancipated, often at the hospital, were buried at the Cemitério do Alto das Cruzes by their own surviving friends. Included among the dead were some Africans who had been freed by the Portuguese colonial authorities, such as local judges and the Tribunal de Prezas.[133] In contrast, in neighboring Benguela human bodies were said to be "covered with only a few inches of earth . . . for the hyenas to dig up and eat what they liked, and then strew the residue about."[134]

In the same period, those recaptured Africans who died of infectious diseases in the El Vedado quarantine buildings near Havana were normally buried in the nearby Cementerio de los Protestantes or in the unconsecrated ground that lay immediately next to it.[135] Just as had been happening in Benguela, during the 1820s, 1830s, and 1840s there were repeated refer-

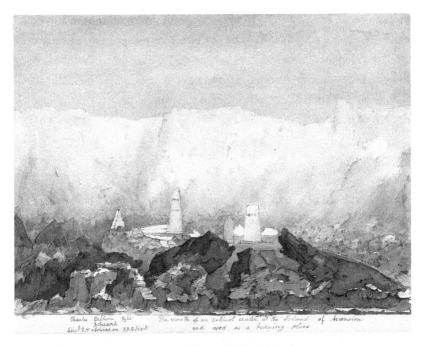

Fig. 19. Bonetta Cemetery. NMM: Album. Art/10. MS65/134.

ences to bodies of bozal Africans that had been interred close enough to the surface to be dug out by passing by dogs and vultures, events that were "terrorizing those who would walk" in its neighborhood.[136] Equally troubling were reports of the bodies of deceased Africans who had arrived at Havana in slave ships being thrown overboard within the harbor and being devoured by fish, a circumstance that led to a debate in the Cabildo of the city, due to concerns about the "prejudice to public health" that the practice could cause.[137] Africans who died elsewhere were often taken to another unconsecrated field located near the Cementerio de Espada, an unwalled space where the bodies were often exposed to wild animals and inclement weather.[138]

Different conditions in each of these Atlantic ports contributed to the various levels of development of medical facilities. Even among those places that played key roles in the battle to abolish the transatlantic slave trade, significant differences existed. Being a British colony, Sierra Leone had

more in common with Saint Helena than with the conditions in Rio de Janeiro, Havana, and other Atlantic spots where recaptured Africans were
landed. What they all had in common, however, were their concerted efforts
to fight disease within colonial or imperial contexts, where the control—or
the illusion of control—of peoples and environments was central to their
dreams of hygienic containment.

The Fight against Disease

Dealing with these deadly and debilitating diseases was a harrowing task
wherever anti-slave trade reception centers were established, and when it
came to fighting disease on the front line, some differences clearly existed
among them. Regardless, some basic common procedures took place in all
ports where courts of Mixed Commission and Vice-Admiralty functioned,
as well as in other centers belonging to other Atlantic powers like the French
and the Americans.

As soon as captured slave vessels arrived at any of these ports, the responsibility for the care of those aboard would be transferred from the prize
officer or the surgeon in charge—sometimes the original ship's surgeon or
one sent from the capturing vessel alongside the prize officer—to the local
authorities. After an initial inspection of the health conditions on every ship,
local authorities would then proceed to separate those Africans and crew
members with infectious diseases from the rest. Following prevalent contagionist beliefs, those who were deemed to be a hazard for the public health
of the local communities were sent to lazarettos or quarantine stations, often
being kept on the same vessels, as the rest were landed and relocated to designated reception areas, and on occasion to places even farther away.[39]

Medical treatment normally began as soon as the sick were separated
from the healthy. The work of health practitioners was fraught with danger
from the moment they boarded these ships. Conditions aboard slave vessels
were regularly appalling, as confinement and overcrowding allowed for the
spread of disease and death among the enslaved. Medical practitioners frequently described these dreadful conditions in their correspondence and in
their personal writings. While answering the set of questions presented to them

by the Sierra Leone Commission of Enquiry sent from England in 1826, John Shower, at the time the surgeon of the courts of Mixed Commission and thus the medical officer in charge of visiting all slave-trade vessels arriving in Freetown, confessed to have "generally found the slaves in an unhealthy state, chiefly afflicted with dysentery, diarrhoea, variola and craw craw."[140] He went on to explain that in his opinion their diseases had been "generated from the vessels being over loaded, long passages, exposure to bad weather and bad food and generally a scanty allowance of water and that of a very bad quality."[141]

Shower's opinion was fully supported by that of William Barry, who had been in charge of visiting slave vessels during 1822 and 1823, until the appointment of Shower to the post of surgeon of the courts of Mixed Commission. In Barry's view, the Africans found on captured slave vessels were generally "in a most miserable condition, in a very crowded state, and from unavoidable circumstances badly supplied with provisions and water."[142] He calculated that "the average of sick" might had been of "about one in five," but that the whole of them were "emaciated and unfit."[143]

Similar descriptions were provided by those who boarded seized slave ships in such locations as Rio de Janeiro, Havana, or Saint Helena. The descriptions provided by Thomas Nelson in Rio de Janeiro, for example, were not limited to the case of the *Dois de Fevereiro*. Before taking another "miserable crowd of liberated Africans" to the *Crescent* in September 1843, Nelson and his colleague William Gunn visited the ship in which they had been carried away from their homelands, the *Vencedora*.[144] Baffled with yet another scene of which "no pen can give an adequate idea," Nelson and Gunn were left astonished by "the smallness of the vessel, and the number of wretched negroes who had been thrust on board of her."[145] In fact, Nelson was barely able to credit his own eyes when he discovered "the different protuberances and anatomical peculiarities of the[ir] bones," which appeared "to be ready to start through the[ir] skin."[146] Left with no other option, Nelson and Gunn had to order the sailors under their command to carry each African in their arms to the *Crescent*, as they were otherwise unable to move. And like the human beings they had enslaved and trafficked, the vessel's crew had been affected by smallpox, leading Nelson to refer to the ship as a "floating Pandora's box."[147]

William Macleay, judge of the Mixed Commission Court at Havana, gave a similar report after visiting the captured slave vessel *Intrépido* in 1828. Not only was Macleay eager to highlight the high mortality and morbidity that occurred in the ship's Middle Passage and upon its arrival, but he also pointed out that the crew had been decimated as well by disease, and that even those who had managed to return alive were in a poor state of health, comparable to that of the men, women, and children they had trafficked across the ocean.[148]

As we have seen, in Havana, Spanish colonial authorities frequently took an active interest in the state of health aboard captured vessels arriving in the port, and they endeavored to assume a number of important responsibilities, such as providing the most appropriate quarantine stations and vaccinating the newly arrived Africans against smallpox. For example, in November 1834, a commission appointed by Tomás Romay, at the time the most respected medical practitioner in Cuba, was put in charge of vaccinating all newly landed Africans, starting with those of the schooner *Carlota*, and of reporting on the state of health on every vessel.[149] The first report of the commission, written by Francisco de Sandoval and Juan Angel Pérez y Carrillo, revealed the agony of the Africans they had examined. Even those who appeared to be healthy, they noticed, "were thin and weak."[150] In addition they found "17 in the ordinary state of diarrhea or cholerina, 5 seriously ill, and 4 in imminent danger in consequence of choleric symptoms."[151] The sufferings aboard seized slave vessels were normally so atrocious that when on exceptional occasions a captured ship arrived with a clean bill of health, as did the brig *Firme* in 1828, the captain and crew were commended for showing "a humane conduct," and an "urgent memorial" in their favor was presented before the Court of Mixed Commission.[152]

Across the ocean, in Saint Helena, medical inspections were also routinely carried out as soon as recaptured Africans began to arrive in seized slave ships. These inspections were habitually followed by a separation of the sick and the healthy, as well as one of "the sexes."[153] That disease was present in most of the vessels arriving at this remote Atlantic island was a foregone conclusion. Between 1840 and 1843, according to George McHenry, smallpox alone had been introduced in Saint Helena seven times in seven ships, "each with numerous patients labouring under that disease."[154] McHenry's own description of one of these vessels, the *Marcianna,* was revealing of the actual conditions aboard these ships. As he was examining the deck, he descended to the forecastle, where he found a small space, "large enough to hold about six people at ease, but which was now filled with fifteen smallpox patients, huddled together, with other accessories of a nature unimaginable and unmentionable."[155]

In other Atlantic locations the situation was no different. For example, in 1837 in a letter addressed to Commodore Peter John Douglas, the collector of customs at Montego Bay, John Roby, recounted the "horrible state of disease and emaciation" prevailing among the Africans seized on board the schooner *Arrogante* whom he had inspected upon arrival, explaining that "the thighs of many were not thicker than [his] own wrist."[156] This case was exceptional in more than one way, as accusations of cannibalism were immediately made by a number of Africans against the Portuguese crew of the ship. Although the accusations were eventually dismissed by British colonial and metropolitan authorities, there was little doubt that this group of Africans had been subjected to the worst possible treatment in addition to the suffering provoked by improperly treated hunger, thirst, and diseases.[157]

For those health practitioners who came into contact with Africans and crews, a considerable level of risk to their own lives and health was always present. Just like other officers related to these reception centers, health practitioners were frequently forced to request permission to escape an almost certain death in these contact zones, and on occasion were infected by the very diseases they were curing. Alexander Stewart, who replaced John Shower in September 1826 as the surgeon to the Mixed Commission courts in Sierra Leone, was compelled to flee the colony less than six months later, fearing for his life.[158] And in Saint Helena, where the activities of practitioners in Lemon and Rupert's valleys were well documented, reports of doctors falling sick were not uncommon. For example, in June 1848, James Rawlins, who was the surgeon in charge of Rupert's Valley, contracted dysentery from a group of Africans he had been treating, and who had exhibited a particularly high mortality. Rawlins battled what he considered a "most severe attack of dysentery" for weeks until he finally recovered.[159] A few years later, in another serious case, one of the supporting members of the medical facility at Rupert's Valley, a Mr. McDaniell, was diagnosed with a very severe case of "purulent ophthalmia," which he had contracted from the Africans he had been treating. As a result, his colleague Henry Hartley wrote of his concern that McDaniell would lose the infected eye.[160]

Working conditions for health practitioners in each of these contact zones' reception centers were almost always substandard. Whereas some doctors in places like Havana and Rio de Janeiro were well paid and recognized by fellow professionals across the Atlantic world as leading authorities in their respective fields, the vast majority of those in charge of receiving and treating newly arrived Africans were ordinary practitioners who were attempting to make ends meet. The nature of their work was dangerous and difficult, as the testimonies of some of them, including James Boyle, Thomas Nelson, Robert Clarke, and George McHenry, attest. In addition, their services were for most of the period badly remunerated. In a letter sent to London in 1824, Edward Gregory supported a memorial written by John Shower requesting an increase in the salary he had perceived for his services "in attending upon the slaves brought to Sierra Leone on Board of slave ships."[161] To Gregory, the "nature of the services performed by him was irksome and disagreeable in the extreme for the unhealthy state in which the slaves attended upon by him are generally brought to this colony."[162] Furthermore, and throwing all his support behind Shower's request, Gregory considered that it was his duty "to bear testimony to Mr. Shower's attention to those unfortunate slaves . . . and his assiduity in executing the orders of the Commissioners in all times and under all circumstances."[163]

Shower's plight was far from unique. Throughout the Atlantic world, health practitioners assigned to these reception centers often resigned or threatened to resign because of salaries they considered meager and the dangers they found themselves exposed to. For example, in 1835, David Scott Meckleham, at the time the Havana Mixed Commission court surgeon, resigned his post, and his replacement, Edward Finlay, followed suit in 1839. Finlay bought a sugar mill in the Havana hinterland and turned himself into a slave planter, after the Foreign Office ignored his repeated complaints about his salary.[164] In Saint Helena, it took only a few weeks for

George McHenry to threaten to resign his post at Lemon Valley due to the lack of supplies and insufficient support he received from Jamestown, and less than three months later McHenry again threatened to resign, as conditions had worsened.[165]

The provision of medical care was undoubtedly one of the pillars of each of these Atlantic reception centers. In spite of these continual setbacks and poor working conditions, as soon as inspections on newly arrived ships were effected and the sick separated from the healthy, medical treatments were started in earnest. Just as slave traders and their associated health practitioners had done in their cities, factories, and barracoons along the African coast, and in the interior on rivers and lagoons, officers and practitioners involved with abolitionist efforts in anti–slave trade reception centers did their best to diagnose, prognosticate, and cure the diseases they confronted.

Beyond their always-pressing needs to sanitize the environment, they needed also, of course, to treat and cure human beings. Although the documents that we have inherited by those involved with the abolitionist efforts in the Atlantic frequently mirror those left by slave traders and their associated practitioners, a number of richer sources, such as memoirs and medical and geographic texts, offer a variety of views on how patients were treated, what sort of medicines were used, and how fragmented medical knowledge circulated in more general terms.

Just as had happened in the illegal Atlantic world inhabited by slave traders, and on the vessels of the British, French, and American navies, medical treatment in each of these centers was administered by a combination of African and non-African practitioners. Treatments combined practitioners' Western and African knowledge with a high degree of ingenuity, often effectively. As the testimonies of officers and health practitioners in charge at each of these Atlantic spots attest, the deaths caused by the Middle Passage did not stop when captured ships arrived in these ports and the recaptured Africans were landed.

A relevant account of the conditions in which Africans usually arrived at any of these posts upon being seized by anti–slave trade patrol vessels comes from Andrew Foulis and James Donovan, who repeatedly dealt with newly arrived Africans in the Gambia in the late 1820s and early 1830s. In a

report sent to London in December 1833, they noted that "the greater proportion of Liberated Africans that are weak and emaciated on their arrival at
the Gambia soon afterward die and . . . many after a longer or shorter residence, fall into the same unhealthy state of protracted suffering linger and
also perish from causes not very dissimilar."[166] In the authors' opinion, these
deaths were the result of long captivity in slave barracoons along the coast
and the terrible conditions the Africans had experience aboard slave vessels.

Unfortunately, the death rates for most of the vessels listed in the *Voyages* database do not include the fatalities that occurred after landing.[167]
This absence is quite significant, as an examination of mortality after landing in some of these sites suggests that in a considerable number of cases,
death took place after the Africans were transferred to quarantine stations,
hospitals, or reception yards, and barracoons. Beyond the overwhelming
evidence easily observable in independent cases, it is possible to offer at
least a general view of the lethal peril of the first days and weeks in places
like Sierra Leone, Havana, and Saint Helena.

In Sierra Leone, for example, between January 1, 1827, and June 30,
1830, the staggering number of 1,620 recaptured Africans died in and
around Freetown. These deaths presumably included all Africans who
were landed after the courts of Mixed Commission condemned the ships
on which they had arrived.[168] More poignantly, the report where these figures were given, almost certainly written by James Boyle, stressed that
"one fifth of the whole number of Liberated Africans settled in the colony
from 1808 to the 30th June 1830" had died, "and that three fourths of the
deaths . . . occurred within the first four months after their arrival through
the . . . diseases generated on board the slave vessels."[169]

In Havana, where the information is sketchier and less reliable, registers
kept between 1824 and 1843 at the Depósito de Cimarrones, where many of
the recaptured Africans—especially those who were not deemed to be particularly sick—were taken, is quite revealing of the real situation for those
men, women, and children who had outlived the Middle Passage, but who
did not manage to survive more than a few days or weeks after reaching Cuba.
Out of approximately 12,000 landed in Havana and processed by the Anglo-
Spanish Court of Mixed Commission in those years, 528, 4.4 percent, died at

the Depósito within the first few days or weeks after landing.[170] It is imperative to stress here that this number refers only to those who were healthy enough to be emancipated, and does not include those who had arrived alive but extremely sick, or those who died in other sites, especially at the barracoons that existed all over the city, at the quarantine buildings in the Vedado area, and on HMS *Romney*. Put together, then, the number of fatalities in Havana during the weeks and months following the arrival of the slave vessels was certainly considerably higher. In Saint Helena, where the figures from 1840 onward are more comprehensive, mortality rates—including all those who had been landed, unlike in Havana—were as high as 31.6 percent between 1840 and 1849, then dropping slightly to 28.8 percent between 1850 and 1863.[171] These figures represent a substantial enhancement of previous mortality estimates for the slave trade in the period, which have so far considered only the deaths occurring during the Middle Passage. The new data deserve a detailed study in their own right, as these initial estimates clearly suggest that the chances of dying from diseases contracted during slave trade transatlantic voyages were substantially higher than what we have assumed until now.

More significant for this study is another revelation originating from these figures, namely, that deaths caused by diseases contracted in the Middle Passage or before continued to occur for weeks and even months after arrival, and not only within the walls of hospitals, barracoons, and yards. That outbreaks of smallpox, almost always associated with the arrival of seized vessels, were common in the villages surrounding Freetown or across the valleys of Saint Helena, is unsurprising when considered in this light.

Medical Care in Anti–Slave Trade Reception Centers

To health practitioners in reception centers throughout the Atlantic, the correct diet was perhaps the first step for the satisfactory recovery of recaptured Africans and crews. In the case of the Africans, a similar diet to that dispensed by the slave traders and anti–slave trade prize crews was often the first choice for those attempting to revitalize them. Food staples considered appropriate to speeding up recovery included but were not limited to jerked beef, farinha, beans, and dried fish, all of which were usually found on board slave vessels in considerable quantities.[172] They were usually confiscated from slave traders by the prize crews and landed along with the Africans, with the sole purpose of continuing to use them in the alimentation of the same men, women, and children.

Once the right diet had been decided upon, authorities and health practitioners began treating the landed Africans. Among the most common ailments associated with the slave trade were the mental disorders often caused by the very experiences of enslavement and transportation in subhuman conditions in the bowels of slave ships. In the range of facilities featured at each of the reception centers discussed in this chapter, mentally ill patients were treated in a variety of ways, following prevailing ideas related to mental health. Both in Sierra Leone and Saint Helena mental patients were often treated at buildings or wards specifically designated for them. Although for most of the time we do not have detailed descriptions of what therapies were used to treat their maladies, it would not be far-fetched to speculate that the same treatments used elsewhere at the time were put in practice across the Atlantic world. Almost certainly, among these would have been the reduction by force of particularly aggressive patients. Other therapies may have been practiced as well, especially bloodletting, a popular medical treatment for a wide range of diseases at the time.[173]

In Sierra Leone, some less conventional attempts of rehabilitation were essayed with recently arrived Africans, especially with those who had given signs of wanting to take their own lives. In 1822, for example, upon the arrival of the Spanish schooner *Josefa,* the judges and surgeon of the Mixed Commission Court decided to do their best to stop many of the Africans from throwing themselves in the sea, as apparently they had planned to do. The Africans were quickly moved to Regent Town, one of the villages founded in the vicinity of Freetown for their reception and relocation, with the intention of reuniting them with "settled residents of their country," in the hope that their conversation would relieve them "from their terrors and put a stop to their desperate designs of self-destruction."[174]

As clinical depression and suicide cases increased across the Atlantic, officers and practitioners in each of these reception centers followed similar therapies, attempting to create the best possible conditions for the recovery of the recaptured Africans. Unfortunately, local authorities in Rio de Janeiro and Havana rarely collaborated in these efforts. As a result, relocation efforts often failed because of the lack of proper attention to mentally ill patients.

As in every other realm within the Atlantic world, fevers were among the main diseases that needed to be confronted. Although typhoid, malaria, typhus, dengue fever, and yellow fever were frequent visitors throughout the tropical and subtropical regions of the Atlantic in the nineteenth century, in Africa, they were particularly common and fatal. Various European settlements in this region, including the Gambia, Sierra Leone, Cape Coast, Monrovia, and Fernando Po, acquired reputations as deadly destinations for all European and American visitors and residents. From Sierra Leone, where the British always had a number of health practitioners in residence, we have some of the best descriptions of how practitioners dealt with these fevers.

Nonepidemic fevers like typhoid, typhus, and malaria seem to have been most common along the African coast, as they were responsible for most of the recorded deaths of Europeans and American visitors and residents. Treatment of these fevers, at least until the mid-1840s, employed the potentially deadly combination of bloodletting, purgatives like jalap or colocynth, and mercurial remedies. Of these, the use of mercury was considered to be vital for the preservation of life. Given in various ways, calomel or mercury chloride was the most popular type of mercurial compound at the time. Even though health practitioners harbored doubts about the extent of the side effects of the use of mercury, they continued to use it throughout the period, as salivation—the main observable result of its use—was considered essential in the recovery of patients suffering from fevers. Questions about its positive effects, however, began to be posed by an increasingly large number of practitioners beginning in the first decades of the nineteenth century.

In 1831, James Boyle, who had been a surgeon on board a Royal Navy vessel before taking over the post of colonial surgeon at Sierra Leone, cited the opinion of a deceased colleague to support his own belief in the "injurious" consequences resulting from the indiscriminate use of mercury.[175] In the mid-1840s, Robert Clarke, himself an advocate of the use of mercury in the treatment of remittent fevers like typhoid, reasoned that its use "bequeaths the patient, as a legacy, a pre-disposition to liver and spleen affections, with a long train of dyspeptic complaints, not to mention carious teeth."[176] More poignant was the opinion of navy surgeon Peter Leonard, who in the early 1830s condemned the use of mercury, which he considered to be inefficacious to fight these fevers. Leonard also criticized fellow surgeons who, in spite of having "glaring instance[s] of [its] failure," before their eyes, continued to use it.[177]

Boyle tells us in detail what medicines he used to treat fever patients in Sierra Leone during the first half of 1828. In January of that year, he treated a twenty-five-year-old sailor for more than a week. The treatment began with a single, large dose of calomel. Subsequently, and in no particular order, the patient was administered repeated doses of calomel, calcined magnesia, barley water, saline effervescent drafts, arrow root, fowl broth, and—once he was considered to be convalescent and out of danger—sulfate of quinine. The same man was given daily sponge baths of cold water and vinegar, had leeches applied to his temples and forehead, had mercurial ointment rubbed on his thighs, was forced to gargle astringents, and was given a purgative enema.[178] A second patient, also treated in January 1828, was first administered a large dose of calomel and then was given Epsom salts, James' powder, opium, and finally sulfate of quinine.[179]

Even medical practitioners like David Francis Bacon, who were up to date with new therapies and who rejected the use of mercury for the treatment of most fevers, instead promoting the use of quinine, continued to resort to mercury in some cases. Bacon, who was appointed colonial surgeon in Liberia in 1836, confessed that only mercury could have any sort of positive effect in the treatment of what he called "the real African fever," or "continuous fever," almost certainly referring to typhoid fever.[180]

Bacon, like most of his contemporaries, was fascinated by some of the properties of mercurial drugs, not least their appearance. Unlike others, however, he refused to use calomel and instead relied on iodide of mercury, which he manufactured himself in his laboratory by mixing iodide of potassium and protochloride of mercury. Bacon, who gave himself credit for being perhaps the first to carry out this chemical experiment in Africa, described these two white powders creating when mixed the "most brilliant red, more splendid than vermillion."[181]

Bloodletting and purgatives were the two other main treatments of choice to fight fevers throughout the Atlantic. As we have seen, slave traders as well as their enemies were fond of both treatments, which they implemented with frequency and urgency. Boyle's narrative includes both as central to the therapies needed to cure patients suffering from fevers, and Clarke confirmed the frequent use of both to treat his patients.[182] James Ormiston McWilliam, who spent time in Sierra Leone and Fernando Po while on his way to the Niger River in the early 1840s, was keen to emphasize how common both treatments were. McWilliam was particularly skeptical of the use of the lancet, which he did not consider to be very useful in West Africa.[183] A few years later, Alexander Bryson was even more critical of what he referred to as the "horror of bleeding."[184]

With the passing of time quinine-based drugs became the main weapons in the battle against malaria, though they were ineffective against other fevers. Quinine solutions appeared frequently in lists of medicines administered by colonial officers throughout the Atlantic alongside calomel, jalap, opium, ipecacuanha, silver nitrate, sarsaparilla, tartaric acid, tinctura digitalis, and gum Arabic.[185] Almost every medical practitioner from Europe and the Americas at the time was likely to use some sort of quinine for the treatment of fevers. Quinine, however, was mostly administered after patients had begun their recovery, as many practitioners considered the drug hard for acutely sick patients to endure. In his notes, Boyle related using it after his patients had entered the remission stage, and Alexander Bryson urged practitioners to wait for the remission of symptoms to begin before dispensing quinine.[186]

As time went by and medical evidence mounted and was disseminated, quinine became an essential drug to fight against malarial fevers. Bacon, for example, considered it to be indispensable for his and his patients' survival in West Africa. He recalled taking over as the main medical authority in Monrovia:

My plan of treatment was simple as the disease itself. I had but one direct remedy for it,—one and the same at all times, in every patient, in whatever stage of the interval or paroxysm. This

medicine was the sulphate of quinine. So long as I had supply
of this article, I never had a day's difficulty with a single case of
intermittent [fever].[187]

By the mid-1840s Bacon was hardly an exception as more and more
health practitioners began using quinine to treat malarial fevers, usually referred to as intermittent fevers. In the 1860s quinine had become so popular
that complaints about its abuse began to appear. The anonymous author of
a book published in 1862 claimed that in Luanda "the sulphate of quinine
had become the base for all treatments," and that people were making "a
frightening consumption" of it.[188]

Treatments for other diseases were similar to those used by slave traders and Royal Navy ships' surgeons. Dysentery, for example, was often
treated with a combination of remedies that included calomel, laudanum,
ipecacuanha, and castor oil, while already in the late 1830s ophthalmia was
successfully treated with silver nitrate, a medicine that Thomas Nelson considered to have "magical effects" after conducting a successful experimental
trial in Rio de Janeiro in 1843.[189]

Smallpox was also attended with great industry. Vaccination efforts
were carried out in practically every anti–slave trade reception center during these years. In Havana, as we have seen, recently landed Africans under
the supervision of the Court of Mixed Commission were immediately vaccinated, just as all Africans arriving at the city's port had been vaccinated
since the early part of the century.[190] In Luanda, those citizens who had
employed recaptured Africans were ordered to vaccinate them within two
years of taking them.[191] This disposition led to frictions between the Court
of Mixed Commission and those citizens who had engaged the Africans, as
the former were often unable to secure the necessary vaccines.[192] Enforced
vaccination in Luanda was nothing short of a widespread experiment, for,
as Samuël Coghe has argued, "neither in Portugal nor in Great Britain, let
alone in Angola, was vaccination compulsory at the time."[193]

Overall, and just as had happened in the rest of the Atlantic, the treatment of often-fatal tropical diseases at each of the anti–slave trade reception
centers was effected through a combination of Western and local informa-

tion and knowledge. The use of Western traditional medicinal products like camphor, jalap, calomel, and quinine was duly complemented by remedies obtained from indigenous African flora and fauna. Professional skills to deal with these various diseases were at times combined to achieve the best results. As we shall see, African knowledge about extracting guinea worms or sand fleas, for example, was more effective than anything European or American practitioners could accomplish while treating the same maladies. Africans' botanical remedies, based on centuries of observation, experimentation, and testing, were frequently accepted and adopted by Western practitioners in reception centers all throughout the Atlantic world during the period, leading to the creation of new Atlantic medical cultures.

Upon his arrival in Freetown en route to Fernando Po in the mid-1840s, Spanish Catholic priest and missionary Jerónimo M. Usera y Alarcón remarked on the important work that the Mixed Commission courts established in that port had been carrying out for years. In his narrative he also referred to the plaque placed at the entrance of the Liberated Africans Yard, and copied verbatim its inscription:

Royal

Hospital and Asylum

For Africans

Rescued from Slavery

By British Valour and Philanthropy

Erected A.D. MDCCCXVII

His Excellency Lieut.te Col.l. Mac. Carthy. Gov.[194]

To Usera y Alarcón, as to many other visitors and residents in Atlantic locations where anti–slave trade reception centers were located, two things were apparent. First, these were cosmopolitan places where peoples from the Americas, Europe, Africa, and beyond came together, some voluntarily and others under bondage, and where they interacted in different ways. Second, in these contact zones, disease was an ever-present frightening entity, of which there were plenty of constant reminders, just like that plaque outside

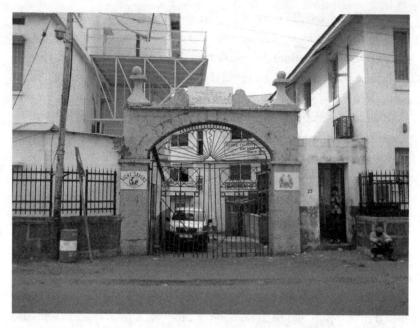

Fig. 20. Liberated Africans Yard plaque in today's Freetown. Courtesy of Richard Anderson.

the Liberated Africans Yard in Freetown, which, incidentally, can still be seen in the same place.

Anti–slave trade reception centers, like slave-trading posts and all vessels involved in one way or another in the slave trade, were at the heart of the contact zones where diseases were endemic and where epidemics could develop suddenly and be unstoppable for considerable periods of time. Although these reception centers did not stop the slave trade, they played a pivotal role in the implementation of abolitionist policies throughout the Atlantic and in the early spread of European colonialism. More significant, in medical terms, they were essential in the ongoing fight against disease, serving as centers for the exchange of medical knowledge.

Likewise, it was thanks to the existence of reception centers that a number of medical facilities, including hospitals—both on the ground and aboard vessels—quarantine stations, and mental wards, were built and developed, allowing for the treatment of thousands of the men, women, and children who otherwise would have faced almost certain death or lifelong disabilities. Of course, these installations also represented an important part of the protocolonial infrastructure needed to foment free trade and Western military expansionism along the coast of Africa.

From identifying to controlling to fighting disease, each of these reception centers and those in charge of running them constituted essential elements in the fight against disease, bequeathing contemporaries and future generations with reams of information that was preserved only because the centers were, unlike anti–slave trade patrol ships, sited on land, where conservation of documents was more likely.

A Shared Struggle

Cooperation, Learning, and Knowledge
Exchange in the Atlantic World

On the other hand, the slave-dealers, in their selection and application
of the large stores of medicines found on board the vessel, may be
presumed to have been guided by some experience of their
beneficial effects.
—Pascoe Grenfell Hill, *Fifty Days on Board a Slave-Vessel*

IN ITS ISSUE of August 4, 1828, the small, outward-looking *Gibraltar
Chronicle and Commercial Intelligencer* featured a peculiarly long extract
from an anonymous letter from Matanzas, Cuba, dated almost two months
earlier. The subject of the missive was the horrifying dengue fever epidemic
afflicting the inhabitants of Matanzas and Havana. The author, probably
one of the many Americans who had settled in the region after 1817 under a
policy of encouraging white immigration onto the island, explained, "speak-
ing literally," that the disease privileged "no age nor color," attacking
all those living in both cities.[1] He described in detail the multiple pains
and aches associated with the malady, as well as the fevers that usually accompanied it. Dengue fever, he wrote, puzzled all those who came into contact with it: "It would be impossible for one who has not been a witness to
the progress of the disease, to form an idea of its effects."[2] How to treat dengue fever constituted an even more bewildering question, as literally nothing that the health practitioners had tried, from orange and lemon juice to

166

cataplasms to the feet, had improved the health of those affected. Finally, and touching on one of the most poignant debates of his time, the writer speculated that dengue fever was a contagious disease; in his view there were "grounds on which to form such an opinion."[3]

To the inhabitants of Gibraltar, a British outpost heavily involved at the time in the British anti–slave trade efforts in the Atlantic, and where a raging yellow fever epidemic was causing havoc at the time, news about a potentially deadly new foe on the horizon was probably alarming.[4] This letter extract also highlights the increasing speed with which news could traverse the Atlantic at the time.[5] Such exchanges of information and knowledge could be, as in this case, between private individuals and governments representing different Western nations and states; among health practitioners employed all over the Atlantic; and between Africans, Americans, and Europeans involved in one way or another with the slave trade or with the efforts to abolish it. In many cases, these interactions generated debates that helped understanding of how these diseases were caused, in what ways they developed, and how they could and should be treated, but more important, they advanced policy-orientated ideas around the best methods for controlling entire populations based on racial stereotyping, and for shaping the manners in which they interacted with non-Western peoples.

In this chapter I scrutinize these exchanges and debates with the intention of offering a comprehensive examination of how knowledge related to diseases and their cures was created and disseminated, as a response to the demands of the slave trade and its abolition, throughout the contact zones of the Atlantic world. I question the ways in which these debates helped disseminating new understandings of various diseases, assessing new therapeutic methods while experimenting with human bodies, and testing new ways of controlling and dominating entire populations. Gaining a deeper understanding of these processes is an essential complement to the discussions vis-à-vis the struggle against disease in the illegal slave trade that have been at the center of this book's previous chapters.

Knowledge Exchanges and Debates in the Slave-Trade
Contact Zones

In the late 1810s and early 1820s, French physician Nicolas Chervin wrote to a number of medical practitioners who had had firsthand experience dealing with cases of yellow fever in the Caribbean and other parts of the Americas.[6] Chervin did not limit his correspondence to practitioners based on French colonies or former colonies, writing also to a number of them in Spanish- and English-speaking American territories, where the transatlantic slave trade was still active. Key to Chervin's concerns was a matter that had puzzled his contemporaries, and that would continue to do so for decades, namely, whether yellow fever was a contagious disease or not.

Chervin, himself a committed anticontagionist, was hoping for answers that would validate his understanding of the disease and how it was transmitted from one human being to another, and that would deny the mainstream belief in the contagious nature of the disease, put forward by British physician William Pym and others. The answers he received, however, were varied and epitomized the uncertainty among the medical ranks about the nature of yellow fever, its particularities in relation to other fevers, and the best ways of managing public policy during a yellow fever epidemic.[7]

Whether the disease was contagious was, however, his main query, and the health practitioners who replied to his request had much to say about it. Bartolomé Segura, a highly reputed medical doctor who had been involved in the first campaign of vaccination against smallpox in Cuba, told Chervin that based on his own understanding of what contagious diseases were—diseases propagated from one person to another, always showing the same symptoms—yellow fever was not contagious, as those who got close to patients suffering from it did not necessarily contract the disease.[8]

Segura's colleague at Santiago de Cuba, Joaquín José Navarro, was of the same opinion, noticing that those arriving from Europe were more likely to get the disease than those who had been living in the tropics for some time and who had been exposed to its ravages on a daily basis. Pointedly, Navarro argued that there was little or no evidence that African slaves who had been arriving in Santiago de Cuba on slave vessels had ever been attacked by the disease. "For what they knew," he wrote, "there was no exact information about whether the vómito [yellow fever] had ever attacked them."[9] Navarro was also keen to indicate, however, that his conclusions were limited by the fact that the very meaning of the term *contagion* was "vague and undetermined."[10]

Both Segura and Navarro were health practitioners in a port city that was an increasingly favored destination for the transatlantic slave trade and where, in the words of British consul David Turnbull, yellow fever regularly committed "the most cruel ravages."[11] As such, they were men who were aware of the diseases of the African coast as well as of those of the Caribbean tropics. Dealing with recently arrived sick Africans, or Europeans, was part of their daily labors. Consequently, their opinions on the matter were taken seriously and incorporated by Chervin into his narratives about the non-contagious character of yellow fever.[12]

Other medical practitioners like Pym, Louis Castel de Vielfoy, and Evariste Bertulus, who had also been in direct contact with yellow fever and other tropical diseases, disagreed to various degrees with Chervin, arguing the case for contagionism and supporting government policies to implement strict quarantine controls across the Atlantic—policies that also supported new colonial outposts and the opening of new markets for the products of the nations they represented. Debates between contagionists and anticontagionists, often politically charged, revolved largely around yellow fever and to a lesser extent to the bubonic plague; they continued well into the nineteenth century and often included discussions about sanitizing human bodies, physical environments, and overall human behavior.

In the late 1840s, there was a particularly vitriolic exchange on this matter between Pym and Alexander Bryson, whose mildly contagionist ideas in *A Practical, Medico-Historical Account of the Western Coast of Africa* failed to impress Pym. By the time of this debate, Pym had been knighted and appointed to the post of superintendent-general of quarantine of Great Britain, making him one of the most important medical authorities in the British Empire. After carefully studying the records of the famous Bulam expedition and its ship *Hankey*, blamed for having created the first Atlantic epidemic of yellow fever in the early 1790s, Pym was the first to offer a clear account of yellow fever—which he called Bulam fever, after the island where the *Hankey*'s colonists had succumbed to it.[13] Over the years, he traveled the Mediterranean and the Atlantic, in charge of implementing quarantines anywhere yellow fever or the bubonic plague struck. He was posted to Gibraltar as soon as yellow fever attacked that British military outpost in 1828.[14] His late 1840s exchange with Bryson—who had been exposed to all the evils of the transatlantic slave trade in Africa for several years—pitted two of the most remarkable and knowledgeable health practitioners of the time against each other, providing a fascinating debate at the end of which the main standing issues left unresolved were whether yellow fever was indeed a particular fever, or just another type of African remittent fever and whether it had a contagious nature or not.[15] Not even well-known stories like that of Robert McKinnal, surgeon of HMS *Sybille*, who was said to have swallowed a whole pint of black vomit from a recently deceased patient in 1830 in order to demonstrate the noncontagious nature of the disease, were enough to settle such a passionate dispute.[16]

The slave trade had been a propitious environment for the circulation of medical knowledge and for cooperation among foes and friends at least since the sixteenth century, as European expansion took place throughout the world. From early on plants and animals also found their way onto ships—frequently slave ships—that crisscrossed the Atlantic Ocean. Some of these plants, for example, also had medicinal properties that had been traditionally identified by those who knew them and who traded them. Others belonged to similar plant genera, and as such were recognized as potentially useful replacements for those that had been used in other parts of the world.[17] Just as diseases had been traded among different peoples during the Columbian Exchange, knowledge and ideas about how to define, treat, and cure these diseases were shared and discussed with the aim of achieving desired ways of hygienic containment.[18]

Additionally, as historian Pablo Gómez has observed, in the early modern Atlantic a series of "objects and substances . . . competed in the same realm with the materia medicas of scholastic medicine," subsequently appearing "in the histories of circulation and exchange of healing materials in the Atlantic."[19] These early exchanges of information and knowledge were carried out by a wide amalgam of health practitioners who hailed from different cultural backgrounds and healing cultures, and for whom "learning from other practitioners became the norm."[20]

Throughout the centuries and up to the advent of Atlantic abolitionism and the resulting ban against the slave trade, health practitioners—and with them, their ideas and their knowledge—continued to circulate in all directions across the ocean, fostering new debates on therapies, practices, and drugs. By the early nineteenth century there was progress in the prevention and containment of such diseases as smallpox, as the widespread introduction of inoculation and vaccination began to transform the ways in which this disease was understood and combated.[21] New drugs derived from plants found in various regions of the Atlantic world became increasingly common among health practitioners, as their effectiveness was observed. By the early 1820s Peruvian bark or cinchona, already taken to Europe by the Jesuits in the late sixteenth century, was found in virtually every compendium of medicines produced in the Atlantic world, as was, for example, *tinctura digitalis* (tincture of foxglove), used to treat heart conditions, and also considered to be an effective relaxant and diuretic medication.[22]

As new drugs were discovered and innovative therapies were tested in the late eighteenth and early nineteenth centuries, exchanges of information and knowledge also continued. Largely as a result of the persistence of the slave trade along the African coast and in the Americas, these exchanges increasingly incorporated opinions and knowledge of non-Western health practitioners, whose firsthand experiences dealing with diseases and illnesses was finally starting to be appreciated by their Western counterparts. These debates and exchanges, no longer limited to health professionals educated in European and American medical schools, took place all across the Atlantic world. Slave-trade contact zones, including slave and anti–slave trade ships, factories, and reception centers, constituted propitious settings for these debates and exchanges to flourish.

For health practitioners, these debates and exchanges were almost always directly associated with various life-or-death personal experiences in the course of their healing work in various regions of the Atlantic. For example, the need to develop practices such as vaccination against smallpox or the fresh questions raised about the efficacy of mercurial and bloodletting treatments were now debated with as much frequency along the coast of Africa as they were in the American regions served by the nineteenth-century illegal trade. These interactions often influenced academic and public discussions that were taking place almost simultaneously in Europe and the Americas, as is apparent from the numerous reports and articles published in medical journals at the time on both sides of the Atlantic.[23] More important, these exchanges and debates also influenced policy, as they unlocked areas of the Atlantic world formerly closed to Western actors, allowing for a gradual increase of protocolonial scrambles, and for the consolidation of European colonies already established along the coast of Africa.

From the first decades of the nineteenth century African practitioners participated actively in these debates and exchanges, even if they were rarely given due credit. Although Western practitioners habitually dismissed their ideas and practices, considering them at best potential apprentices to supposedly more advanced medicine, on some occasions they were interviewed and listened to, and their knowledge was incorporated into the broader medical knowledge of the time. Whereas debates and exchanges sustained in these contact zones were much better documented when the participants were European or American health practitioners, the voices and knowledge of their African counterparts sporadically found their way into the historical record, gifting us with much valuable information about a neglected side of the story of medical debates and exchanges in the nineteenth-century illegal slave trade. As slave traders and their foes tussled for spheres of influence in Africa, the resulting process of cooperation and learning helped shaping the ways in which diseases were understood, remedies and therapies applied, and further forms of Western expansionism devised and refined.

Cooperation, Learning, and Mistrust

During his visit to the Bight of Benin in the mid-1840s British explorer John Duncan came across a town where smallpox was, in his own words, making "dreadful havoc."[24] Although Duncan was not a health practitioner himself, he seems to have been familiar with the methods of cowpox inoculation, which he recommended to the locals so that they could stop the disease from taking more victims. In his narrative, Duncan mentioned that the local sheikh, once shown this technique, was immediately willing to give it a try, and for that reason commissioned his "doctors, of whom he [had] a great number," to learn the new method.[25] In another case, William H. Hole, the surgeon of the British merchant ship *John Cabot,* commented that upon his arrival in Cape Mount in October 1838, the "natives" upon being informed that he had some medical knowledge, came immediately requesting "Fitish" from him, in order to cure their maladies.[26]

Stories like Duncan's and Hole's, reflecting a supposedly accepted superiority of the white man over the Africans, were commonly found in both travel accounts written during the period and documents produced by Western practitioners and authorities along the coasts of West, West Central, and East Africa. Chronicles like these emphasized the perceived supremacy of Western medical knowledge in diverse ways, contrasting it with the absence of knowledge, superstitious beliefs, and "savage" practices Western practitioners had observed among the Africans they had met. Even to those who were in charge of implementing the abolition of the slave trade in these contact zones, Africans continued to be condescended to and described with racist epithets, while their medical knowledge was rarely regarded as anything but backward and ineffective.

The numerous records left by the British, the French, the American, and other Western powers along the African coast during these decades provide a testament to habitual denigration of Africans' medical knowledge and practices. John Smith commented in 1851, for example, that "the African doctor in the exercise of his craft, gulls the people almost as much as the priest does in exercising his."[27] Smith went on to mock the rituals that accompanied medical therapies, in particular their dances and the way they dressed before administering treatment.[28] Other European and American visitors to various African regions in this period provided equally contemptuous accounts. French explorer and officer Gaspard Mollien, who was for a short time in charge of the French hospital at Gorée Island, considered the medical knowledge of the marabouts along the coast of Senegal limited to "the application of a few simple remedies, or to the composition of certain charms written on paper, which they make their patients burn and drink the ashes."[29] In their narrative of their visit to the Bights in the early 1830s, Richard and John Lander took this disdain even further, referring to health practitioners as "idle, lazy fellows who pretend to be Mahomedan priests," and to all medicinal derivatives from local roots and plants as "inefficacious" and "altogether useless."[30]

Western health practitioners, authorities, and neighbors also complained frequently about being the subject of derision whenever they tried to treat sick Africans. Mary Church commented that in Sierra Leone liberated Africans who had spent some time in the colony demonstrated "prejudice in favour of their country doctors and old women."[31] Also in Sierra Leone, William Ferguson commented in 1831 that his patients had the "habit of having recourse to native practitioners and their mode of treatment."[32] In the same vein, Ferguson's colleague John Bell noticed that when the Africans thought that they would "require a length of time for their cure," they would "retire to the country to procure the herbs and different medicines prescribed for them by the native medical men" instead of seeking his advice.[33] In an even harsher report written in 1830, James Boyle was quick to blame the African dressers who had been in charge of liberated African settlements in the neighborhood of Freetown for causing avoidable fatalities due to their "ignorance."[34] Boyle blamed this "Quackery in country medicine" for the death of a missionary catechist residing in the village of Kissy, adjacent to the liberated Africans hospital.[35]

This perceived lack of knowledge and skills led Superintendent of Liberated Africans Dixon Denham to request from governor Hugh Lumley the appointment of "some European medical officer to superintend the native dressers who are now resident in each village," as he did not consider native practitioners—in this case he referred to a Mr. Brown, who was in charge of the Kissy hospital—of being capable of taking care of large numbers of sick people.[36] To be sure, Denham's concerns were nothing new, as only three years earlier the colony's deputy inspector of hospitals and principal medical officer, J. A. Schelky, had encouraged weekly visits to the liberated African villages located around Freetown in order to "estimate and to stimulate the vigilance of the dressers attached to these villages," as he did not trust them to dispense the necessary medical treatments in the absence of a Western practitioner who could supervise them.[37]

In the best cases, Western practitioners often saw their African counterparts as feasible pupils to whom they could pass on their "superior"
knowledge of the diseases they were confronted with, and their allegedly
most effective cures. Such an educational enterprise, however, was not always as straightforward as they desired it to be, as their prospective disci-
ples were not always ready to engage with foreign practices that in many
cases were highly questionable. Regardless, some Western practitioners like
Robert Clarke were keen to impose their medical knowledge upon their
subordinates. Remarkably, Clarke suggested delivering "regular lectures on
surgery and the practice of physic at the Hospital to intelligent Creoles,"
with the intention of removing the "deep rooted prejudices" that prevented
Africans "from seeking efficient medical assistance."[38]

From the early years of the Sierra Leone colony, the British had sent
local youngsters to England to acquire training in various professions. At
least one of them, John Macaulay Wilson, the son of the ruler of Kafu Bul-
lom, returned to Sierra Leone sometime around 1800 and worked first as an
apothecary, and subsequently as an "acting surgeon to Regent" in charge of
controlling an outbreak of smallpox in 1817, and as the "assistant colonial
surgeon posted to the Hospital at Leicester" in 1822.[39] By the mid-1820s,
Governor Neil Campbell had also appointed two maroons named William
Brown and Ibert "to the hospital and the pharmacy."[40]

Although hardly ever acknowledged, African practitioners, in fact,
collaborated more and more with their Western counterparts as the years
went by, contributing their own knowledge, innovations, and skills to the
identification and treatment of disease. Reception centers, for example, allowed for a combination of African and Western remedies, which were at
times recorded and discussed by American and European officers, residents, and visitors. Western knowledge often engaged with local botanical
expertise, as physicians who had graduated from Oxford, Edinburgh, and
Yale universities, gave credit and/or questioned the therapies and drugs of
their fellow African practitioners.

Although it was not unusual for African practitioners to be blamed for
the failure of treatments, at times they gained a reputation for working wonders
in curing diseases for which Western practitioners had no answers. For every

vilification of their faculties—like the one against the African practitioner in charge of the garrison at McCarthy Island in the Gambia River, accused by Thomas Eyre Poole, of being an "illiterate Black quack"—there were examples of Africans whose knowledge was recognized and admired by their Western counterparts.[41] Prominent among them was the celebrated Dr. Saguah, who in his youth had been a slave to the African Company at Cape Coast castle. Over time and after receiving his freedom in 1822, Dr. Saguah was said to have "learned to compound medicines," and to have stayed as a member of the medical department at the hospital, perceiving a small salary.[42] Dr. Saguah was said to be well respected and trusted, and his reputation in the late 1830s "stood so high that he was frequently consulted on the diseases of the climate in preference to medical gentlemen from Europe."[43]

George McHenry, in Saint Helena, also recognized the contribution made by "several Negroes at the Hospital" in Lemon Valley since he had begun working there.[44] McHenry was especially keen to highlight the role of one of them called João, who did "a great deal of the offensive work at the hospital." So much so, he argued, that he requested from the island's government that João's name should be struck down from the liberated Africans register, and that he should be awarded "a salary of 1 shilling a day" for his hard work.[45]

Official recognition also came from local authorities. A number of descendants of liberated Africans received medical education in England and Scotland in the mid- and late 1850s, then returned to Sierra Leone to exercise as health practitioners. Among them were a James Africanus Beale Horton, an Ibo; George Theodore Manly, a Wolof; and William Broughton Davies, an Aku (Yoruba). All three exercised their profession with success from the moment they returned to the colony and until their deaths, but Horton left a longest-lasting legacy. Horton, educated at the University of Edinburgh, was perhaps the first African to state to the British government the need for a tropical medical school in West Africa.[46] Horton also gained celebrity for his writings, which included some medical texts and the classic *West African Countries and Peoples,* published in 1868, in which he defended Africans against racial stereotypes frequently attached to them by Western visitors to Africa.[47]

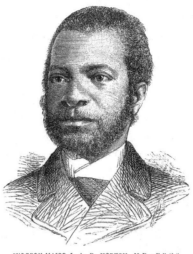

SURGEON-MAJOR J. A. B. HORTON, M.D., F.R.G.S.
An African Doctor on the Army Medical Staff
Born 1834 ; Died Oct. 15, 1883

Fig. 21. Africanus Horton. *The Graphic. An Illustrated Weekly Newspaper.* December 29, 1883, issue 735.

Horton demonstrated that the myths about superstitious beliefs of the Africans and their rejection of Western medicine were often distortions of actual events resulting from the racial prejudices of visitors who looked with contempt on anything they consider inferior and backward. The stories told by Duncan and Clarke also had the unintended effect of proving that African health practitioners beyond European and American settlements were often keen observers and eager learners of new medical therapies, to the benefit of their patients. In fact, all along the African coast other health practitioners were not only willing to share their knowledge but also eager to learn about new medicines and treatments. The introduction of the vaccine against smallpox in particular seems to have been particularly successful almost anywhere that Western practitioners took it.

Slave-ship masters and slave dealers frequently shared vaccines against smallpox, and the British and the French in their colonial enclaves along the shore also introduced vaccines with the aim of arresting the spread of the disease and of bolstering their own overseas operations and ventures. Vaccination efforts, for example, often brought African practitioners to the forefront of ongoing discussions. In West Africa, local residents in and around European settlements, or in those places explorers visited occasionally, seem to have adopted the vaccination method with little hesitation. According to Niger Expedition physician James Ormiston McWilliam, the mallams he encountered in his voyage up the Niger were "delighted when the protective power of vaccination was explained to them."[48] Until the arrival of the vaccine, several African peoples had relied on the method of inoculation, as well as on local botanical remedies to treat those who had contracted it. Robert Clarke left perhaps what it is the only description from this period of how recaptured Africans in Kissy treated those who were infected with smallpox: "The Liberated African lubricates the body of the patient laboring under small-pox, with palm or nut oil, the patient nesting close to the fire, which is always kept burning, during the progress of the complaint."[49]

By the mid-nineteenth century vaccination was widespread throughout the Atlantic world and was being adopted by all those involved with the illicit slave trade. In Cuba, since the early part of the century, health practitioners had made a point of vaccinating—or inoculating when vaccines were not available—as many slaves arriving from Africa as they were able to.[50] In Brazil vaccination was taken just as seriously. Maria Graham, while visiting the southeast of the country in the early 1820s, noticed that local practitioners would travel to nearby plantations to vaccinate the slaves at least once a year.[51] She also pointed out that the "vaccine establishment formed in Brazil in 1804 having declined, it was renewed both at Bahia and Rio, and immense numbers of persons of all colours were vaccinated."[52] Equally, in Angola, by the late 1840s, Mixed Commission judges tried to keep enough vaccine to vaccinate every liberated African within a period of two years, something that had been a common practice in Sierra Leone at least from the mid-1820s.[53] In Africa, where smallpox was a permanent affliction, learning this new preventive method meant that many lives—often the lives of those sent into the transatlantic slave trade—could be saved. McWilliam's account of his vaccination crusade as he moved from one place to another in West Africa offers palpable proof that far from being indifferent, Africans were excited to hear about the positive effects of the vaccine and enthusiastic to be vaccinated and to learn how to vaccinate themselves. In addition to the eagerness of the mallams to learn the method, McWilliam reported that women in Egga and Nupe "unhesitantly brought their children on board to be vaccinated," and in several other locations local health practitioners "were shown the operation and instructed how to perform it."[54] All in all, McWilliam concluded: "Had it not been for the disasters that befell our expedition, I had great hopes of the extension of vaccination throughout the Niger, by means of the Mallams."[55]

These exchanges were not, however, always smooth. Disagreements and mistrust between Western and African health practitioners were almost certainly common during the period, although they were not always recorded. On one occasion, a Portuguese anti-slave trade squadron crew member wondered, almost in comical fashion, "where the Cabinda doctors and many other [doctors] in Africa went in search of Aesculapius's staff, I have not been able to find out."[56] One of these few instances of disagreement was documented by George Thompson in the mid-1850s, when his attempts to treat an epidemic of measles with European remedies met stern resistance from Mendi "country doctors," whose opinions regarding the best course of action to arrest the disease differed diametrically from those of Thompson.[57] Thompson recounted that he had eventually prevailed by showing his Mendi counterparts the "superior success" of his Western method, a circumstance that led many to bring "their children to the Mission house for treatment."[58]

William F. Daniell, perhaps better than any other Western health practitioner to visit Africa during the period of illegal slave trade, was able to leave detailed descriptions of the status and knowledge of treatments and medicinal remedies of his West African counterparts. Daniell, who had been calling on various regions of West Africa since at least 1838, wrote extensively about every medical matter he encountered. Many of his articles, in which he gave extensive credit to the medicinal properties of African plants, appeared in the *Pharmaceutical Journal* between 1849 and 1865. In these written pieces he introduced Western audiences to a number of African botanical remedies resulting from such well-known staples as the kola nut, and others partially or completely unknown like the Katemfe or "miraculous fruit of Soudan," as well as the poisonous properties of the cassava root and other plants.[59]

In his *Sketches of the Medical Topography and Native Diseases of the Gulf of Guinea, Western Africa,* published in 1849, Daniell also discussed the important role of health practitioners, cataloguing the terms used for them in the regions he visited: "Lock-a-Mallaku, Benin; Gangur or Gangam, Kongo; Maïmahgané, Haussa; Ebbebok, Old Calabar; Jarrahlah, Mandingo; Enishogung or Ologung, Yarruba; Dey-yo, Kroo; &c."[60] In some cases, Daniell was able to provide accurate and detailed accounts of the role of practitioners, their sex, and their responsibilities. For example, he noted that in "the Ebo country adjoining the river Andony," health practitioners were divided by sex. The male ones were called dibia woca and the female dibia wy. Daniell also noted that dibia wy were mostly concerned with performing circumcisions, while their male colleagues usually treated a wide array of diseases and maladies.[61]

Daniell's main contribution, however, was his unusually exhaustive description of African seeds, roots, shrubs, fruits, and flowers used for medicinal purposes by the peoples he came in contact with. He described multiple seeds, like those of the Cassia or *Senna occidentalis* (coffee senna) treasured by the Wolof in the Senegambia, and the *Piper guineense* (Guinea pepper), used "as an adjunct to allay the irritative effects of cathartic and other medicines."[62] He also described a number of other plants such as the common watermelon, which in his words was "highly esteemed by the natives for its antiseptic, refrigerant and antifebrile effects," and the Baobab fruits, used to make poultices to treat "rheumatic and other painful afflictions of the limbs."[63]

Finally, on occasion, Daniell described how the men and women he encountered in his travels prepared certain medicinal remedies. He described, for example, the manner in which "one of the most efficient and valuable tonics that had hitherto been classed amongst the catalogue of native medicines" was prepared in the Bight of Biafra. He wrote that the locals would roast the fruit of the *Raphia vinifera* (soap berry) in a slow fire in order to separate the "cortical pulp from the nut which encloses," subsequently heating the resulting substance until it lost its "intense astringency." Daniell suggested that in the absence of quinine, he had regularly used this tincture "in combination with other indigenous carminatives" to treat those who were suffering from "loss of appetite and frequent vomiting" after "prolonged attacks of remittent fevers, and with the best results."[64]

Although Daniell's acknowledgment of the botanical knowledge of the African health practitioners he met was unusually thorough, others who visited various parts of the continent, often due to their involvement with the slave trade or its abolition, left fragmented accounts about this marvelous pharmacopeia. Notable among this literature were a travel account by Lyons McLeod, the British consul at Mozambique in the late 1850s, the little known Portuguese relation by Francisco Travassos Valdez, and the foundational work of British physician Thomas Winterbottom.

Lyons McLeod arrived in Mozambique in 1857, and during his time in Eastern Africa wrote profusely about the cultures and peoples he met in the region.[65] In his two-volume *Travels in Eastern Africa; with a Narrative of a Residence in Mozambique,* he carefully reported on a number of medicinal plants and roots found on the northern mouth of the Zambezi River, and how they were employed by inhabitants from the town of Tete "in the treatment of the diseases" they were exposed to.[66] Among the long list of herbs and compounds described in detail by McLeod were remedies against ophthalmia (mucorongo or jambalão root); bubos and gonorrhea (root of mupumpua); and chest pains (infusions of musequesse leaves and a poultice obtained from mupanda-panda). To treat fevers they used a decoction made out of the bark of tussi, to which the Banyans seemed to attribute "the same effects and virtues of cinchona."[67] According to McLeod, another efficacious remedy against the fevers were the heated and dried leaves of chirussa, which were also used to treat cases of tenesmus.[68]

Travassos Valdez, the son of the first Count of Bomfim, was a Portuguese traveler and writer who left works recounting his travels throughout the African continent. His attention to the ways in which the Africans he met treated various diseases and maladies resulted in a number of descriptions that complement those left by others like Daniell, McLeod, and Winterbottom. While visiting the kingdom of Kazembe in the late 1850s, he observed that its inhabitants were able to extract remedies against the diseases that affected them from "their vegetable productions," also noticing that they could "often succeed in making wonderful cures."[69] While describing Ambaca, in today northwestern Angola, he mentioned that "the district abounds with shrubs, herbs, and roots of a medicinal nature, many of which are considered very valuable."[70]

Travassos Valdez gave an even more compelling description of these medicinal remedies and their effectiveness when he discussed how they were produced and used in the locality of Calumbo, in the outskirts of Luanda. Some of the most widely used of these "efficacious" remedies were:

> Muamua, an antidote for diarrhea; mussanda, used for headaches; quibato, applied for pains in the limbs; vua; muondongolo, given to children as a vermifuge; dendo, for jaundice; catalango, used as a gargle for sore throats; mufixi, used as an anodyne, and as a vermifuge; mufungambo and musangola, both used for pains in the stomach; and quicununo, applied to heal wounds.[71]

Winterbottom, whose narrative was written around six decades earlier at the turn of the nineteenth century, not only identified a number of diseases such as sleeping sickness and lymphatic filariasis but also often emphasized the curative properties of various African plants and roots. Long before Daniell had done so, Winterbottom described the astringent properties of the kola nut and the *Nauclea sambucina,* which was used to treat diarrhea and dysentery.[72] While discussing other West African treatments for dysentery, he nominated as "their most celebrated remedy," one which deserved "more particular attention from Europeans," the bark of bellenda or *crossopteryx,* which was either mixed with boiled rice or served as a strong infusion.[73]

Winterbottom also praised the skills and knowledge of his West African colleagues. In fact, he even mocked European criticism of African superstitious beliefs, reminding his colleagues that similarly ridiculous superstitions had been common in Europe only a short time before.[74] Winterbottom also admitted something that virtually no other Western practitioner of this age did, that "considerable pains" had been taken "to discover those [African] remedies upon which the natives place their chief dependence for the cure of diseases."[75]

Other travelers left less detailed accounts of African health practitioners' skills and knowledge of botany. Among them was the previously mentioned John Smith, who after mocking several African practitioners, admitted that some of them were indeed capable of administering what he called "medical measures" that included treating feverish patients with palm oil unguents and jalap.[76] Likewise, a crew member of the Portuguese anti–slave trade squadron vessel *Conde de Vila Flor* pointed out during a visit to Cabinda that illiterate local doctors relied on "a stick with a coiled snake" and "witchcraft and divination" in their practice of medicine. Sneering aside, he acknowledged that Cabinda practitioners knew the medicinal "uses of several plants, and were able to use them to treat various diseases."[77] James K. Tuckey and Christen Smith also left a description of the use by inhabitants of Inga, a town along the Congo River, of "infusions and decoctions of native plants," including "a species of dioscorea," to prevent diarrhea and dysentery.[78] While recalling his visit to Africa, John Duncan was similarly keen to point out that along the Grain Coast, malaguetta was "an important article in the materia medica of the native doctor, being used both as a stomachic and external irritant."[79] During his discussion of the role of health practitioners in this part of the coast, Duncan concluded that the "deyâbo," professional men who combined "the medical and priestly office in the same person," were skilled in the use of medicines, and that they would always give their "undivided attention to one patient at the time."[80] Later in his narrative, while discussing medical practices in southern Guinea, Duncan concluded that certain African individuals had "the art of curing certain diseases," and that they would "make no pretensions to any further knowledge of the art of medicine."[81]

No wonder Winterbottom himself was eager to point out that Africa, though long neglected, had "in store for future observers some articles which [could] become important acquisitions in the materia medica."[82] From Joseph Hawkins noticing the astringent properties of the relatively common guava fruits in 1797, to Joshua Carnes raving about the multiple properties of pineapple more than five decades later, ultimately it became apparent that the same continent that frightened Westerners with deadly diseases also offered ways to remedy those maladies.[83]

Out of Africa, the medical knowledge and skills demonstrated by Africans were also recorded on occasion. One of the keenest observers and witnesses of these abilities and knowledge was George McHenry, the first health practitioner to be put in charge of the liberated Africans reception center and hospital in Saint Helena in 1840.[84] In the published account of his time in Saint Helena, McHenry referred to "the knowledge possessed by the negroes respecting the art of healing," declaring this knowledge "more considerable than Europeans would be inclined to give them credit for."[85] To McHenry, many of the Africans who had worked alongside him trying to palliate the suffering of recently arrived Africans "were intimately acquainted with the medicinal qualities of plants and other articles employed in their pharmacopeias." Among these, he enumerated a list of remedies with "purgative, emetic, astringent, diaphoretic, and epispastic medicines."[86] McHenry also gave credit to the Africans he met in Lemon Valley for their acquaintance with the method of inoculation to combat smallpox, and noticed that they were experts at bleeding, an operation they would normally carry out "by means of scarifications made with a knife, over which is applied in a horn in which the air is rarified and exhausted by suction."[87] Finally, McHenry was quick to point out that the African healers also had certain clinical skills, and that they were capable of performing amputation surgery "remarkably well."[88]

Exchanges of knowledge between Westerners and Africans happened all along the African coast, on African islands like Saint Helena, and into the interior of the continent for as long as the illegal slave trade continued. Among the many treatments that Western practitioners attempted to learn from their African colleagues was extraction of guinea worms. Numerous Western health practitioners and travelers noticed that the "natives" in Africa were much more proficient at extracting the worm intact, avoiding the extended suffering imposed on the patient if the worm was broken into pieces, as commonly occurred. Clarke and Bryson both discussed the guinea worm and praised the skills of African practitioners in extracting it, an opinion also shared by Charles W. Thomas, who commented in the early 1860s that the expert "native manipulators" would normally "take the process out of nature's hands" by "making an incision through the skin, over the middle of the worm," and then extracting it "by a single traction."[89]

Cooperation and learning also occurred among Westerners who visited or settled in Africa. For example, in the Portuguese colony of Bissau, complaints about the lack of medical supplies, facilities, and practitioners filled page after page of contemporary letters and reports sent to Lisbon and the Cape Verde islands. These letters highlighted the colonists' dependence on informal collaboration with practitioners and other officers belonging to friendly European powers in the region.[90] According to Joaquim Antônio de Mattos, governor of Bissau in 1830, these supplies, facilities, and practitioners were indispensable if the settlement was to survive and thrive in the face of deadly diseases and constant attacks from the neighboring Africans.[91] Although responses to these pleas did not always meet the required standards, these requests were indeed addressed by the Portuguese authorities, which had built a hospital and a pharmacy and had provided the additional practitioners.[92]

In a more explicitly illustrative case, the fortuitous visit of a Portuguese health practitioner resident in Luanda to Saint Helena in the late 1840s allowed for one such exchange to take place on the origins and best treatment for another disease rarely discussed anywhere but in the South Atlantic, that of *mácula*, or *bichu du cu*.[93] In one of the best reports on the therapeutic courses of action thought to be most effective against this potentially lethal disease, Manuel Maria Rodrigues Bastos, a Portuguese doctor and the surgeon-general at Luanda, observed to his British counterpart that the disease was frequent among the Africans, especially among those from Congo and Moxicongo. He described the symptoms as a flux accompanied by a "dilatation of the anus, ulceration and sometimes with worms," with feces characterized by a very particular smell.[94] Since the medicines that would normally arrest the advance of dysentery and diarrhea had little impact on this malady, Rodrigues Bastos proposed pursuing empirical and experimental treatments. His suggestions included giving the patients "an enema of gunpowder, agua ardente [brandy] or Eau de Cologne and . . . added Lime juice."[95] The opinion of Rodrigues Bastos about this "the most horrible disease that carries off great numbers of the Negroes" was confirmed by James Rawlins, the surgeon at Rupert's Valley, a year later in another letter, also addressed to John Young, the local collector of customs.[96]

A similar instance of collaboration was reported in the mid-1840s by Spanish Catholic priest and missionary Jerónimo Usera y Alarcón upon his arrival at the island of Fernando Po. Soon after his landing at Port Clarence, Usera y Alarcón was welcomed by several missionaries, including health practitioners William Newbegin and G. K. Prince, to whom he referred as a surgeon and a medical doctor, respectively. Usera y Alarcón praised both men, especially Prince, who, in his own words, "not only lent us gratuitously the assistance of science with the greatest attention, but also gave us in the same manner the most expensive remedies from his medicine chest, preparing them with his own hands."[97]

During his cruising off the coast of Mozambique, William Owen also reported occurrences of collaboration among the Europeans who had settled along the coast with the aim of participating in the illegal slave trade. Remarkably, Owen found that Europeans residing in Quelimane had "condemned altogether the treatment adopted by European surgeons," and were instead relying on remedies and treatments used by "the oldest inhabitants amongst their countrymen, or [those] of the blacks."[98] He wrote that they had given up completely on bloodletting or the use of mercury, and that their "favourite medicines" were "Peruvian bark, Columbo root, rhubarb, and the Marrello pill."[99] He made a similar observation while visiting Mozambique, noticing that "the only remedy used by the natives" was Peruvian bark, and that bleeding had been completely abandoned.[100]

Unsurprisingly, perhaps the only slave dealer of this period to leave a testimony of the work of African practitioners was Theodore Canot. In his narrative he referred to their work more than once, at times questioning the ways in which they mixed superstition with dubious preparations that he considered harmless homeopathic remedies.[101] On at least one occasion, however, Canot described the abilities of a renowned West African "native doctor," who prescribed that he "be cupped in the African fashion" by scarifying his back and stomach, and then applying plantain leaves to the resulting wounds.[102] Other Western health practitioners confirmed Canot's description of the efficiency with which this West African healer was able to bleed him. Notably, James Young, who was an assistant surgeon in the British army, informed the Commission of Enquiry led by Major Rowan in 1826 that he had begun bleeding his patients "by cupping the temples in the native manner," making it clear that he considered this technique to be effective.[103]

Exchanges beyond the African Coast

As Africans were forcefully relocated on the American side of the Atlantic, either as slaves or after being recaptured by anti–slave trade patrols, they took with them their botanical and medical knowledge and skills and reproduced them in their new environments. As an understandable result, such interactions as had been taking place along the African coast also occurred in places as diverse as Brazil, Cuba, the West Indies, and the United States. The resulting fragmentary evidence, dispersed across such wide and diverse geographical areas is sketchy, as historian Sharla Fett has noted, "can only be interpreted in general terms."[104]

Perhaps the best proof of the transfers of such knowledge and skills to the Americas can be found in the herbal remedies and healing practices associated with religions such as Candomblé in Brazil and Santería in Cuba, which continue to be broadly practiced in these cultures.[105] It is not a coincidence that most recorded allusions to such knowledge and skills come from Brazil and Cuba, the two places in the Americas that continued to receive African slaves until the 1850s and 1860s, respectively.

In both Brazil and Cuba, Africans were able to find numerous familiar plants. Some were closely related to those they had known in their African regions of origin, while others had traversed the Atlantic at some point during the more than three hundred years of exchanges that had taken place since both continents had become interlinked by the slave trade.[106] According to Carney and Rosomoff, while Africans would also have come across a vast array of plants that were entirely new to them, many others "would have been recognizable because they belong to plant genera found in both the Old and the New World."[107]

Certainly African practitioners had been at work in the Americas from a much earlier period, as various historians have pointed out in the past few years.[108] This was the case in Brazil since at least the late seventeenth century, according to James H. Sweet, who described a few relevant cases, including that of Lucrécia, an Angolan slave, who in 1680 was offering medical attention by giving herbal remedies to fellow slaves, while also performing a *calundús* in Bahia.[109] More recently, Pablo Gómez has recounted the case of Francisco Mandinga, an African healer living near Cartagena de Indias in 1664, who was said to have used his knowledge of herbal remedies to treat and cure a number of people in the small town of Coloso.[110] In a similar fashion, while examining the interaction between French and African health practitioners in eighteenth-century Saint Domingue, Karol K. Weaver was able to identify a variety of enslaved practitioners who, while embracing to a certain extent Western medicine, also continued to use their African knowledge to treat those under their care. Among these practitioners were the *hospitalières, infirmières,* and *accoucheuses,* or hospital caretakers, aides, and midwives respectively; the *gardiens de bêtes,* or veterinarians; the herbalists; and the *kaperlatas,* who were often considered as sorcerers.[111]

It is not far-fetched, then, to assume that daily interactions between African and Western health practitioners were a common occurrence throughout the nineteenth century in the American regions most affected by the transatlantic slave trade. On occasion, during the first few decades of the century, a number of references to African remedies as well as healing practices and practitioners were recorded in Cuba. In 1844, for example, Pedro Gangá, an enslaved African in the jurisdiction of Guamutas, east of Matanzas, was said to have bought an ounce of ingredients that when put together would help him cure his gonorrhea. Among those ingredients were various roots, honeybee, and snails.[112]

A few years earlier, Italian physician and sugar plantation owner José Leopoldo Yarini described a number of charms used by the slaves on his estate to protect themselves from diseases such as cholera. Yarini, a keen observer who showed an unusual interest in the cultural and social practices of the Africans enslaved on his plantation, noticed that some of these charms, including snails, dried weeds, cock spurs, and seeds of Palma Christi, were occasionally used as medicinal remedies.[113] After inquiring about the use and effectiveness of these remedies and charms, Yarini shed light on another aspect of this African botanical knowledge and its transplantation to the Americas, that of "the evil herbs that other Negroes use[d] to kill people."[114] As a matter of fact, the same Pedro Gangá, who was said to have bought the ingredients for a remedy against gonorrhea in 1844, was accused, alongside fellow African Jacobo Lucumí, of poisoning Juan Bautista Després, the owner of the sugar mill Unión. Several witnesses, including a number of slaves, stated that they had blended the poisonous ingredients into Després's coffee, leading to his almost immediate death.[115]

Western health practitioners and travelers living in or visiting Brazil also recorded instances of African medical knowledge transplanted to the Americas, as did some local authorities on occasion. Cases of poisoned masters, as João José Reis has pointed out, were not unusual in Bahia during the period, with arsenic sulfide and a number of "Herbs and roots known to African medicine" often being employed.[116] These herbs and roots, of course, were also used to treat and cure various maladies and diseases. For example, in 1849 George Gardner left a short account of *curadores* in the region of Minas Gerais "who apply remedies with many mysterious ceremonies."[117] Although Gardner never mentioned the origins of these practitioners, it is plausible to infer that at least some of those he met were African or of African descent. Decades earlier, in the 1810s, Henry Koster also referred to the healers he found in his travels, noticing how they were able to use a vast array of medical remedies obtained from the plants and roots they had access to. Notable among them were the *ipecacuanha branca* and *ipecacuanha viola,* both used as purgatives, and the *herva cobreira,* used to treat snakebites.[118] While discussing the origin of the latter, Koster was keen to point out that every time he had seen the plant, its specimens had been "carefully preserved in a pot."[119] To Koster, this was a clear indication that the plant was not indigenous to Brazil. In fact, he wrote, he had been told "that it had been brought from Africa."[120]

Beyond the importation of botanical knowledge, Africans taken to Brazil frequently shared their healing skills. Sangradores, many of them African born, were common across Brazil during the first half of the nineteenth century.[121] In 1856, British-American traveler Thomas Ewbank published an account of his experiences in Brazil after spending the previous ten years in the South American empire. In his narrative, Ewbank recalled that bloodletting

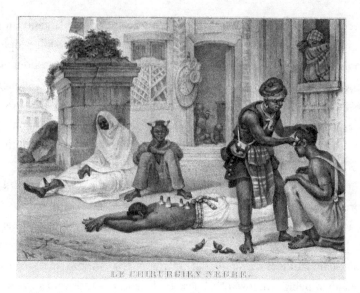

Fig. 22. "The Black Surgeon." African health practitioner in Rio de Janeiro. Jean Baptiste Debret, *Voyage Pittoresque et Historique au Bresil* (Paris: Firmin Didot Frères, 1834–39), vol. 2, plate 46.

or cupping was "a favorite African remedy," which was expertly done by Africans and their descendants in the places he visited, although with a "process and apparatus . . . of extreme antiquity."[122] He observed that the "operator scratches the skin with a flint, places the wide end of a sheep's horn over it, and sucks out the air."[123] This treatment, in his opinion, was usually performed in the sunshine, as those who performed it insisted that its effects were "then most beneficial."[124]

The bloodletting or cupping skills shown by Africans in this period were recorded in other parts of the Americas too, notably in the United States, where a navy officer in charge of a number of Africans taken from the Spanish ship *Castilian* in 1860, noted in the ship's log that an African woman had been "making gashes with a razor on the swollen feet of a scurvy patient," a procedure that he found consistent with contemporary Western medical practices.[125] Another known case was that of José del Sacramento, a native of Peru and a professional bloodletter on board the slave brig *Negrito*, seized and taken before the Mixed Commission Court at Havana in 1832.[126]

In one of the most detailed descriptions of the work of African health practitioners in Brazil, Robert Walsh's book *Notices of Brazil in 1828 and 1829* offered a number of portrayals of these men and women at work on the American side of the ocean. Walsh, too, made a passing reference to their bloodletting abilities, recalling that they always used cupping to treat rheumatic pains.[127] Almost immediately after this observation, he pointed out that "'negroes" were always the operators in charge of bloodletting patients, as they were too for extracting the *bichu*, or guinea worm. Echoing descriptions by those who had observed this procedure in West Africa, he remarked that they "dexterously, with the point of a blunt knife, raise the skin and open the flesh round the sore, without drawing blood or breaking the sac; and thus extract the whole nidus without disturbing a single egg."[128]

Walsh also described Africans' *bolsa das cobras*, or snake bags, in which they carried the ingredients needed to prepare remedies against a number of maladies, including snake bites and chest pains. To treat the latter, Walsh observed, the African took "a joint of the [snake], pounded it in a mortar and collecting some herbs, he boiled them together." A few spoonsful of these, he said, was sure to relieve the most obstinate attack.[129]

In what it was, perhaps, Walsh's most noteworthy reference to transferences of skills, he recalled that one of his friends had given up on Western medicine to treat a severe case of sciatica. He had relied on the faculties of one of his African-born slaves, who, standing on the patient's back and hips, trampled him "with his naked warm feet." The treatment, although painful, was so successful that "in a short time the pain entirely ceased," no doubt a result of the "rough, but effectual mode of negro champooning."[130]

The narratives left by Walsh, Ewbank, Koster, and others illustrated a continuous process of exchange between Africans and Westerners in Brazil and other parts of the Americas after 1807. Practitioners interacted and learned from one another, each at times bowing to the resources and efficacy of the ideas and therapies of the others.

Upon visiting Quelimane in the late 1850s, perhaps the most famous African explorer and Christian missionary of the nineteenth century, David Livingstone, described the herbal remedies he had observed at this slave-trading port during his visit. Livingstone, like others before him, saw the potential that African plants and roots could have on the materia medica of his day: "It might be worth the investigation of those who visit Africa to try and find other remedies in a somewhat similar way to that in which we found quinine."[131] Western visitors and residents in the diverse regions of Africa involved and affected by the transatlantic slave trade were, just like Livingstone, exposed to lethal and debilitating diseases—and to the local remedies formulated to treat them. From 1807 and until the effective abolition of the human trafficking in the mid-1860s, Westerners and Africans came across each other in the slave-trade contact zones, not just in Africa but throughout the Atlantic world. It was in these spaces that diseases, and the ideas and remedies to treat and cure them, were exchanged.

Whereas mutual mistrust and suspicion often permeated these contacts, there is evidence of a level of engagement and cooperation that went beyond the oversimplified view of Western practitioners as all-righteous, know-it-all physicians who imparted wisdom wherever they went. In fact, as we have seen, African practitioners also shared their knowledge of remedies, cures, and medical procedures with their Western colleagues, who often embraced that learning and shared it with a wider audience.

Cooperation, however, was not only about exchanging fragments of knowledge but about working together, often giving due recognition to the work of those who were in the front line of the fight against disease. Although cases of meteoric rise to positions of power or influence, such as that of Dr. Saguah at Cape Coast, were rare, Africans did join medical corps in almost every Atlantic spot affected in one way or another by the slave trade. As Andrew Pearson has revealed, George McHenry, after spending long and continuous periods of time working side by side with African practitioners who had arrived in Saint Helena on slave trade vessels, "developed considerable respect for their capabilities as healers."[132] In another contemporary account, William Whitaker Shreeve, who in the 1840s spent six years in Sierra Leone working for the courts of Mixed Commission, acknowledged the skills of the "African dressers and compounders" who worked under the supervision of Dr. William Aitkin in their local village hospitals offering basic care.[133] Shreeve also commented on the work of Africans at Kissy hospital, where there were "a pharmacopist head and assistant African dressers, nurses, etc."[134] Robert Clarke, too, made an important reference to the skills shown by some Africans he met in Sierra Leone, who were able to concoct an emollient potion to treat rheumatism by processing the fat and bones of chimpanzees.[135]

Through decades of daily interactions Western and African practitioners formed opinions of one another, and based on the relationships they developed, they were able to exchange their knowledge and to debate, often as equals, approaches to the diseases they were forced to confront. Although the role of Africans in these exchanges has usually been "presented in the negative, through lack of cooperation, willful or otherwise," the historical record, especially when examined from a circumatlantic comparative scope, categorically reveals a very different story.[136] A story in which African practitioners did not passively accepted the white man's ideas and knowledge, but one in which they engaged, shared, challenged, and contributed to what can only be described as debates that took place day to day, in the field, and over many years, and that resulted in the implementation of new medical philosophies and therapies, and in the discarding of obsolete ones.

Closing Remarks

Beware, beware of the Bight of Benin, for few come out, though many go in.
—Old anonymous rhyme

ON DECEMBER 14, 1833, the brig *Negrito* entered the harbor of Havana, having been seized by HMS *Victor* off the coast of the island of Tobago three weeks earlier, while carrying 526 Africans embarked at the port of Ouidah.[1] Upon its arrival in the Cuban capital, a report of the health on board the ship noted that during these three weeks a total of 36 Africans had died of various diseases, in spite of the attention and care given to them by the surgeon of the *Victor*, John West.[2] The mortality and the morbidity on the *Negrito* were not out of the ordinary. If anything, this was a vessel where death and disease had not materialized in their worst incarnations.

The relatively mild image conveyed by the paperwork of the Anglo-Spanish court of Mixed Commission and the Spanish authorities, however, contrasts sharply with a watercolor depicting the Africans on the vessel's deck, painted by French traveler François Mathurin Adalbert, Baron of Courcy, who happened to be visiting Havana at the time.[3] Through Courcy's eyes, the scene on the deck was just as Dantesque as that described by Thomas Nelson while examining the *Dois de Fevereiro* years later in Rio de Janeiro. Courcy's watercolor reveals the extreme anguish and pain of the Africans who had crossed the Atlantic in the hold of this slave ship.

Although Courcy's painting only shows the deck of the *Negrito*, by looking at the watercolor one can imagine how much poorer conditions belowdeck may have been. The scene presents a considerable number of Africans—around seventy by my count—lying about the deck, visibly suf-

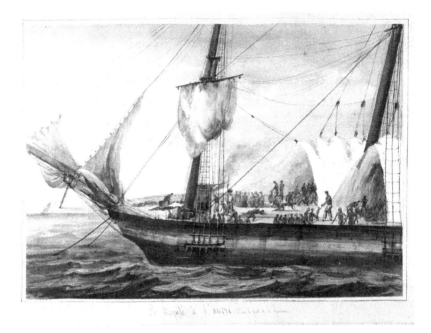

Fig. 23. *Negrito*, Havana. Baron de Courcy. Courtesy of Eduardo Uhart.

fering from fatigue and disease. Others can be seen crawling or prostrated in obvious discomfort, while many are hiding under the customary tents put up by the British crew to protect them from the sun and the rain.

The comparison between the written and graphic evidence pertaining the *Negrito* serves to highlight some of the main issues and themes that have been discussed in this book. Even though the ravages caused by the diseases of the slave-trade contact zones were not exceptional in the case of the *Negrito*, there is little doubt that the situation faced by all those involved in this slave-trading expedition was dire. The visual representation of their suffering by a firsthand witness serves as a reminder that even the most accurate reports by those critical of human traffic in the Atlantic may have frequently failed to reveal to a real extent the horrors of the slave trade, especially in those cases that were not considered to be particularly calamitous.

The struggle against disease in the slave-trade contact zones took many shapes and forms, and resulted in a transformation of medical cultures across the nineteenth-century illegal Atlantic world. Preventive measures that included moral policing and the sanitation of diverse environments were central to a dream of hygienic containment that also hid an expansionist agenda. Some of these measures, notably the bills of health and the implementation of quarantines, were applied with the double intention of stopping diseases from spreading and of furthering protocolonial goals, including territorial expansion, control of colonized populations, and advantageous access to new markets. Additionally, new experimental treatments, often lethal, were part of the fight against slave-trade diseases.

Although this was a period in which medical experimentation and discoveries led to new understandings of endemic and epidemic diseases, it would be erroneous to define this battle only via Western medical practices and their occasional breakthroughs, or through the actions of Western practitioners alone. Instead, as I have made clear, the struggle against disease within the slave-trade contact zones was in fact determined by the combined knowledge and action of health practitioners from different backgrounds, including Africans and their descendants in the Americas. Just as European and American health practitioners on both sides of abolition applied and shared their knowledge within the slave-trade contact zones, African practitioners did the same. Sometimes their pharmacopeia was ridiculed, by ignorant Westerners clinging to prejudice and stereotypes about "uncivilized" Africans. But the surgical strategies and medical knowledge of African practitioners, and especially their medical use of local plants, came to be recognized and adopted by many of their Western counterparts.

The one thing that slave traders, anti–slave trade personnel, and Africans involved in one way or another with the slave trade or its abolition had in common was their need to control diseases that hindered their activities throughout the Atlantic. Disease was their common adversary, a mortal foe that could strike any time along the coast of Africa, in the middle of the Atlantic, or in cities and plantations on the American side of the ocean. The evidence uncovered and examined in the pages of this book strongly suggests that irrespective of who they were, health practitioners in the slave-trade contact zones had access to similar medicines and knowledge to fight against these diseases. There is enough evidence to argue that they also shared with one another any fragmentary knowledge they acquired during the period.

The work of health practitioners was dangerous. They were in frequent contact with people who had been infected with a variety of diseases. Many practitioners lost their lives in Africa, at sea, or in the Americas, fighting the transatlantic slave trade or serving it. Some used their time in the slave-trade contact zones to experiment and try new treatments and medicinal combinations, some of which proved just as lethal as the very diseases they were fighting. Their passionate debates about contagion—leading one anticontagionist to the extreme gesture of drinking the vomit of a dying yellow fever patient—and their embrace or rejection of questionable therapies like the use of mercurial drugs or bloodletting highlight their doubts and their ingenuity. Londa Schiebinger has persuasively argued that some practices within the slave-trade contact zones—particularly those of Western practitioners—were "not purely scientific" but did embody "questions fired in the colonial crucible of conquest, slavery, violence, and secrecy."[4]

There is enough qualitative and quantitative evidence as well to assert that in the post-1807 slave trade, illegal practices led to an increase in the human suffering. As Walter Rodney maintained decades ago, the intensification of slave trade–related warfare in many areas of the African continent unquestionably raised "the number of people killed and injured so as to extract the millions who were taken alive and sound" onto the Atlantic.[5] Long terms of residence in barracoons along the African coast and hurried shipping practices, necessary to avoid capture by anti–slave trade cruisers, were commonly cited as causes of increased mortality during the period. More to the point, deaths that occurred after arrival in places like Sierra Leone, Saint Helena, Brazil, and Cuba—a considerable number, according to the fragmentary information we have—should be factored into the mortality figures associated with the slave trade after 1807.

All in all, the story told in these pages is one of familiarity and strangeness among people who converged in the slave-trade contact zones, a story of vulnerability and strength in the face of difficulty. The anxiety and concerns provoked by the illegal character of the slave trade shaped responses to disease across the board for all those involved, ushering in new medical cultures, and contributing to the dissemination of fragmentary medical knowledge among friends and enemies. From Captain Owen's empirical assumptions about a possible link between mosquito bites and fevers to Dr. Saguah's medical proficiency on the Gold Coast; from the repeated doubts about the use of mercury and the lancet raised by anti–slave trade patrol surgeons like James Boyle and Peter Leonard to the many descriptions of African practitioners expertly dealing with guinea worms, fevers, and other maladies, the unremitting human struggle against diseases in the slave-trade contact zones had a shared and cooperative dimension.

Although the results of this struggle were diverse, there is little doubt that these health practitioners categorically changed the ways in which diseases were tackled, as they also changed Western approaches to Africa as a potential place to conquer, colonize, and exploit. While I have not set out in this book to prove the progression of medical knowledge over time, I would be negligent not to conclude with an acknowledgment that resulting medical practices enabled and encouraged Western imperialism throughout the Atlantic in decades to come. That "honor" should fall to Robert Clarke, a firsthand witness of these events during the 1830s, 1840s, and 1850s, to whom by the mid-1850s West Africa no longer appeared as "an object of terror."[6] Thanks to "better housing, dressing, temperance and quinine," Clarke remarked—at once allaying the fears of his kind and further encouraging their colonialist aspirations—as the transatlantic slave trade reached its final years, the region could no longer be called "the white man's grave."[7]

Notes

Introduction

1. Nelson, *Remarks on the Slavery and Slave Trade of the Brazil,* 44.
2. Ibid.
3. Ibid.
4. Ibid., 46.
5. Ibid., 45.
6. Ibid.
7. Ibid.
8. The surgeon of the *Crescent* at the time was Dr. William Gunn; Hautain, *New Navy List,* 218.
9. This second vessel was probably the Brazilian ship *Asseisseira,* also captured by Lieutenant Foote. Ouseley to Captain Jones, Senior Officer. British Legation, Rio de Janeiro, February 24, 1841; and Ouseley to Lieutenant [Malachi] Donellan. British Legation, Rio de Janeiro, February 24, 1841. TNA: Foreign Office 84/364. For the dreadful conditions found on board the *Asseisseira* upon capture, see William Morris to David Morgan. HMS Partridge, Rio de Janeiro, January 14, 1841. OUWL: Thomas Fowell Buxton Papers. Sections A–B. Mss. British Empire s. 444 (27).
10. Of the 180 only 160 survived the journey to Berbice, and soon after arriving, four more died. Deposition of Gabriel Johnston, Berbice, May 26, 1841. TNA: Foreign Office 84/438.
11. Ouseley to Palmerston. Rio de Janeiro, August 7, 1841. HCPP: 1842 [403] Correspondence with Spain, Portugal, Brazil, the Netherlands, Sweden, and the Argentine Confederation, relative to the slave trade. From January 1 to December 31 1841 inclusive (Class B), 703–4.
12. Crosby, "Virgin Soil Epidemics." See also Kiple, *The Caribbean Slave* and "Mortality Caused by Dehydration."
13. In a recent book Londa Schiebinger has argued that in the eighteenth century Caribbean slaves were not treated as guinea pigs as one would have expected, but that they were considered as property that needed to be protected. Nineteenth-century slave traders frequently took a similar approach across the

Atlantic, attempting to keep as many enslaved Africans alive and in good health as possible, in the hope of maximizing profits; *Secret Cures of Slaves,* 7.

14. LoGerfo, "Sir William Dolben and 'The Cause of Humanity' "; Garland and Klein, "Allotment of Space for Slaves"; Engerman and Eltis, "Fluctuations in Sex and Age Ratios"; and Haines and Shlomowitz, "Explaining the Mortality Decline."

15. Eltis, *Economic Growth and the End of the Transatlantic Slave Trade.* Among the most recent in-depth studies of the conditions on slave ships during the eighteenth century see Stephanie E. Smallwood, *Saltwater Slavery: A Middle Passage from Africa to American Diaspora* (Cambridge: Harvard University Press, 2008); Eric Robert Taylor, *If We Must Die: Shipboard Insurrections in the Era of the Atlantic Slave Trade* (Baton Rouge: Louisiana State University Press, 2009); and Sowande' M. Mustakeem, *Slavery at Sea: Terror, Sex, and Sickness in the Middle Passage* (Urbana: University of Illinois Press, 2016).

16. Voeks, *Sacred Leaves of Candomblé;* and Carney and Rosomoff, *In the Shadow of Slavery.*

17. Vaughan, *Curing Their Ills,* 2. This topic is further discussed by John K. Thornton in *Warfare in Atlantic Africa,* 7.

18. Curtin, *Death by Migration,* xiii, 1–2.

19. Gómez, *The Experiential Caribbean,* 133.

20. Crawford, *The Invisible Enemy* and *Deadly Companions.*

21. Although the Dolben Act provisions that regulated the slaves-to-tonnage ratio in any slave voyage had to be renewed on an annual basis, they were finally made permanent in 1799 by the new Slave Trade Act of that year. See Cohn, "Deaths of Slaves"; and Steckel and Jensen, "New Evidence."

22. Crosby, "Infectious Disease and Demography," 125. See also Thornton, *Africa and the Africans,* 142–43.

23. Crosby, *The Columbian Exchange.*

24. Reperant, Cornaglia, and Osterhaus, "Understanding the Human-Animal Interface," 65.

25. Following Pratt's lead, I use Fernando Ortiz's concept of transculturation as a documented phenomenon that took place in the slave-trade contact zones throughout the period studied in this book. See Pratt, *Imperial Eyes,* 6; and Ortiz, *Contrapunteo cubano,* 93–97.

26. Pratt, *Imperial Eyes,* 6. See also Barros and Stilwell, Introduction to *Public Health and the Imperial Project;* and Gómez, *The Experiential Caribbean.*

27. See also Curtin, *Disease and Empire;* Cook, *Born to Die;* and Graden, *Disease, Resistance, and Lies.*

28. Crosby, "Virgin Soil Epidemics," 299.

29. The very title of this book, which presents yellow fever as a demon, is one of the many cases where these comparisons have been made.

30. Contagiousness was in itself a central issue, debated by physicians for most of the nineteenth century. Debates between contagionists and anticontagionists often centered around diseases such as cholera morbus, bubonic plague, and yellow fever. As a matter of fact, the very definition of contagion was the subject of intense debates in the period; Tulodziecki, "From Zymes to Germs." See also the debates provoked by the publication of William Pym, *Observations upon the Bulam Fever,* which raged well into the middle of the nineteenth century.

31. Clarke, "Short Notes on the Prevailing Diseases," 74.

32. A ward for mentally ill patients was established at Kissy in the 1820s to treat mostly patients who had been psychologically affected by the horrors of slavery and the Middle Passage. In 1854, Kissy's upper hospital was turned into a "lunatics' asylum." Clarke, "Short Notes on the Prevailing Diseases," 64. See also Akyempong, Hill, and Kleinman, *The Culture of Mental Illnes,* 28.

33. Schliesinger, *Sacred Cures of Slaves.*

34. Reperant, Cornaglia, and Osterhaus, "Understanding the Human-Animal Interface," 65–66.

35. AOHCH: Actas de Cabildo Trasuntadas, Book 9, fols. 436v–437v (February 6, 1637).

36. Ibid., Book 14, fols. 457–459v (September 16, 1667); Book 15, fol. 133 (April 10, 1676).

37. Brown, *The Reaper's Garden,* 258.

38. Jensen, "Safeguarding Slaves."

39. Peruvian bark had been in use across the Atlantic since the seventeenth century, but it was not until the mid-nineteenth century that practitioners turned it into the most important drug to fight these fevers. Kiple and Kiple, "Deficiency Diseases in the Caribbean," 199–200; Pearson, *Distant Freedom,* 177–79; and Crawford, *The Andean Wonder Drug,* 47–53.

40. See, for example, Newson and Minchin, *From Capture to Sale,* 247–71.

41. Gómez, *The Experiential Caribbean,* 43–44.

42. Linebaugh and Rediker, *The Many-Headed Hydra,* 14–15.

43. Ibid., 328–29.

44. Ibid., 158.

45. See, for example, Ross, "The Career of Domingo Martinez"; and Barcia, "Fully Capable of Any Iniquity."

46. Perhaps the most notorious case, and certainly one of the earliest, is that of English physician and abolitionist Thomas Winterbottom, *An Account of the Native Africans in the Neighbourhood of Sierra Leone.*

47. See, for example, Sheridan, "The Guinea Surgeons on the Middle Passage"; Steckel and Jensen, "New Evidence"; Haines and Shlomowitz, "Explaining the Mortality Decline"; Klein, Engerman, Haines, and Shlomowitz, "Transoceanic Mortality"; and Smith, *Ship of Death*.

48. Among this small number, see Eltis, "Fluctuations in Mortality"; Barros, " 'Setting Things Right' "; Graden, *Disease, Resistance, and Lies;* Pearson, *Distant Freedom;* and some of the chapters in Pimenta and Gomes, *Escravidão, doenças e práticas de cura no Brasil.*

49. Games, "Atlantic History and Interdisciplinary Approaches," 168-69.

50. See, among others, Savitt, *Medicine and Slavery;* Sheridan, *Doctors and Slaves;* Weiner and Hough, *Sex, Sickness, and Slavery;* Curran, *The Anatomy of Blackness;* Bankole, *Slavery and Medicine;* and Paugh, *The Politics of Reproduction.* For a discussion on the cis-Atlantic term see Armitage, "Three Concepts of Atlantic History," 16, 23-28.

51. Pimenta, "Barbeiros, sangradores e curandeiros no Brasil,"; and "Entre sangradores e doutores"; as well as Santana and Santos, "Sangradores Africanos na Bahia do Século XIX"; Graden, *Disease, Resistance, and Lies;* Nerín, *Traficants d'ànimes;* Rodrigo y Alharilla and Chaviano Pérez, *Negreros y esclavos;* and Barcia, *Una sociedad distinta.*

52. Propositions of this sort are not a thing of the past. For example, in February 2018 British historian Mary Beard created a Twitter storm when she wondered "how hard it must be to sustain 'civilised' values in a disaster zone," while discussing the sexual exploitation scandal that followed the actions of Oxfam staff in Haiti. See https://www.tcs.cam.ac.uk/news/0038460-mary-beard-sparks-twitter-outrage-over-oxfam-scandal-tweet.html.

53. See, for example, Palmer, "From the Plantation to the Academy"; Weaver, *Medical Revolutionaries,* 116; Hogarth, *Medicalizing Blackness;* and Voeks, *Sacred Leaves of Candomblé.*

54. See, for instance, Chateausaulin, *El vademecum de los hacendados cubanos,* first published in 1831; Imbert, *Manual do fazendeiro ou tratado doméstico;* and Chernoviz, *Formulário ou guia médico.*

55. Kelly, *Old World and New,* 91-93.

56. Murphy, *Metaphor and the Slave Trade,* 130.

57. Boyle, *A Practical Medico-Historical Account;* and Davies, *Extracts from the Journal.*

58. Boyle, *A Practical Medico-Historical Account,* v.

59. Davies, *Extracts from the Journal.* See also The William Davies Letters (viz. letters written by the Rev. William Davies, 1st ("Africa") prior to his appointment as a Missionary to Sierra Leone, 1814. NLW: Cyf., 24, 1969.

60. Sanneh, *Abolitionists Abroad;* Mouser, "Continuing British Interest"; Tyler-McGraw, *An African Republic;* Huillery, "The Impact of European Settlement"; Everill, *Abolition and Empire;* Ryan, " 'A moral millstone' "; and Grenouilleau, *Quand les Européens découvraint L'Afrique intérieure.*

61. For two relevant cases—both Catholic priests—from Cuba and Brazil in this period, see the writings of Juan Bernardo O'Gavan in 1821 and Leandro Rabelo de Castro in 1842. Barcia, *Seeds of Insurrection,* 80; and Lima, "Como se Cuba não existisse," 240.

62. Ouseley, *Notes on the Slave-Trade,* 25. Smallpox epidemics in Brazil resulting from slave-trading expeditions were nothing new at the time. See Arden and Miller, "Out of Africa." See also Thornton, *Africa and the Africans,* 157.

63. Ouseley, *Notes on the Slave-Trade,* 51.

64. Jameson, *Letters from the Havana,* 2.

Chapter 1. "A Beautiful Spot for a Grave"

1. José Camps to the Marquis of Casa Yrujo. Freetown, Sierra Leone, August 21, 1819. AHN: Estado, 8030, No. 74.

2. Ibid.

3. Bridge, *The Journal of an African Cruiser,* 187. For similar descriptions of the lush vegetation surrounding Freetown see, for example, Samuel Bacon to Smith Thompson. Sierra Leone, March 9, 1820. BL: African Squadron Letters. Vol. 1. 1819–23; and Ricketts, *Narrative of the Ashanti War,* 189–91.

4. Extract of a Dispatch (No. 13) dated Freetown, Sierra Leone, September 20, 1828, from Mr. Smart to the Right Honourable Lieutenant General Sir George Murray, 30. HCPP: Sierra Leone. Return to an Address of the Honourable House of Commons, dated May 19, 1829.

5. Response of Mr. Bell to questionnaire sent by the Commissioners of Enquiry. St. Mary's, Gambia, June 24, 1826. Sierra Leone Commissions of Enquiry. Vol. 2, Appendixes B and C. TNA: Colonial Office, 267/92.

6. Response of William Ferguson. Sierra Leone, April 24, 1826. Sierra Leone Commissions of Enquiry. Vol. 2, Appendixes B and C. TNA: Colonial Office, 267/92.

7. Charles Hoffman to Mahlon Dickerson. Salem, July 26, 1836. BL: African Squadron Letters. Vol. 4. 1829–41.

8. See, for example, Curtin, "The White Man's Grave"; Kiple, *The Caribbean Slave;* Paugh, *The Politics of Reproduction;* Schiebinger, *Secret Cures of Slaves;* and Senior, *The Caribbean and the Medical Imagination.*

9. Jameson, *Letters from the Havana,* 59.

10. See, for example, Graden, *Disease, Resistance, and Lies,* 70–74.

11. Ibid., 73.

12. Paugh, "Yaws, Syphilis, Sexuality," 227.

13. Audouard, "Mémoire sur l'origine et les causes de la fièvre jaune."

14. Carvalho e Menezes, *Demonstração geografica e politica,* 59–61. See also entries from February to April 1839. AHM: Bergantim Audaz/1/12. Diário Náutico (1821–51).

15. Andrés de Zayas, Anastasio Carrillo, Juan Cascales y Ariza and José María Chacón y Calvo to Captain General Mariano Ricafort. Havana, April 9, 1833. ANC: Asuntos Políticos, 35/47.

16. Pratt, *Imperial Eyes,* 6.

17. See, among many others, Hallett, *The Penetration of Africa;* Temperley, *White Dreams, Black Africa;* Lockhart, *A Sailor in the Sahara;* Quella-Villéger, *René Caillié, l'Africain;* and Grenouilleau, *Quand les Européens découvraint L'Afrique intérieure.*

18. Francis Augustus Collier to J. W. Croker. HMS Sybille, St. Helena, March 28, 1830. TNA: Admiralty 1/1.

19. In an analogous case, Commodore Charles W. Skinner, the commander of the U.S. African Squadron, lamented that the diseases associated with the unit's work alongside the coast of Africa had left most of the vessels of his fleet without enough lieutenants to cope with the demanding task they had at hand. Skinner to John Y. Mason. USS Jamestown, Porto Praya, February 19, 1846. BL: African Squadron Letters. Vol. 6. 1845–46.

20. Paugh, *The Politics of Reproduction,* 13.

21. Bashford, *Imperial Hygiene,* 1.

22. Barnes, "Cargo 'Infection,' " 93.

23. Even so, health practitioners like William Fergusson suggested that fevers could also appear in dry and barren landscapes, bringing into question the validity of the miasma theory; Fergusson, *Notes and Recollections,* 89–96.

24. Boyle, *A Practical Medico-Historical Account,* 6.

25. Journal of Her majesty's Sloop "Rapid," Mr. Edward Heath surgeon. Between the 1st January 1847 and the 31st December 1847. TNA: Admiralty, 101/116/4.

26. Adams, *Remarks on the Country Extending from Cape Palmas to the River Congo,* 202; Journal kept by Ernest de Cornulier. French Navy, 1822–23. NMM: LOG/F/4.

27. Joseph C. Miller has suggested that the term probably derived from the word "carneiro" or burial urn; Miller, *Way of Death,* 384, note 13.

28. Pinto de Azeredo, *Ensaios sobre algumas enfermidades,* 48–49.

29. Valdez, *Six Years of a Traveller's Life,* 1: 264.

30. Jameson, *Letters from the Havana,* 59.

31. George McLaren's Naval Journals. Port Royal, July 31, 1835. CUMC: MS Add.9528/2.

32. Andrés de Zayas, Anastasio Carrillo, Juan Cascales y Ariza, and José María Chacón y Calvo to the Count of Ricafort. Havana, April 9, 1833. ANC: Asuntos Políticos, 35/47.

33. Bell to James Rowan. Saint Mary's, Gambia. June 24, 1826. TNA: Colonial Office, 267/92.

34. Response of William Ferguson. Sierra Leone, April 24, 1826; and Response of Alexander Stewart. Surgeon to the Forces. Freetown, November 4, 1826. Sierra Leone Commissions of Enquiry. Vol. 2, Appendixes B and C. TNA: Colonial Office, 267/92.

35. "General Remarks." Journal of Her Majesty's Sloop "Ranger." West Coast of Africa Station. Mr. Constantine Keenan, surgeon. Between 1st January 1861 and the 31st December 1861. TNA: Admiralty, 101/132.

36. Von Zütphen, *Tagebuch einer Reise,* 16.

37. Clarke, *Sierra Leone,* 95. Sunstrokes were often reported throughout the slave-trade contact zones. See, for example, Henry R. Solomon to John Young. [Rupert's Valley], March 30, 1841. SHGA: Colonial Secretary's In Letters, 8 (1840–41). In this missive, Solomon reported one such case and requested "straw hats or caps" from the Saint Helena's collector of customs to supply those working during the day on the islands' roads.

38. Trobriand, *Une aventure de Négrier,* 15–16.

39. "General Remarks." Journal of Her Majesty's Sloop "Ranger." West Coast of Africa Station. Mr. Constantine Keenan, surgeon. Between 1st January 1861 and the 31st December 1861. TNA: Admiralty, 101/132.

40. Response of Dr. Young. London, March 26, 1827. Sierra Leone Commissions of Enquiry. Vol. 2, Appendixes B and C. TNA: Colonial Office, 267/92.

41. Fernández de Madrid, "Memoria sobre la disentería en general," 389.

42. Findlay to George Murray. Sierra Leone, January 3, 1841. SLPA: Liberated African Department Letter Book, 1830–31. No. 4.

43. Burton, *Wanderings in West Africa,* 1: 170.

44. Chalhoub, "The Politics of Disease Control"; and Kodama, "Antiescravismo e epidemia."

45. Audouard, "Mémoire sur l'origine et les causes de la fièvre jaune."

46. For a list of published articles discussing Audouard's theories from the 1830s through the 1870s, see Chalhoub, "The Politics of Disease Control," note 21. For a specific analysis of his work in Brazil, see Kodama, "Dr. Audouard in Barcelona."

47. Allen and Thomson, *A Narrative of the Expedition*, 1: 447.

48. M. C. Perry to the Secretary of the Navy. USS Macedonian, Port Praya, May 17, 1844. BL: African Squadron Letters. Vol. 5. 1843–45.

49. Ibid.

50. For Dr. Reid's ventilation plans and for the purifying chamber at the center of the system, called "the medicator," see McWilliam, *Medical History of the Expedition to the Niger*, 255, 262.

51. Temperley, *White Dreams, Black Africa*, 51.

52. Sigaud, *Du climat et des maladies du Brésil*. See also Rodrigues, *De Costa a Costa*, 306, 352, 367; and Graden, *Disease, Resistance, and Lies*, 73–74.

53. "General Remarks." Journal of Her Majesty's Sloop "Ranger." West Coast of Africa Station. Mr. Constantine Keenan, surgeon. Between 1st January 1861 and the 31st December 1861. TNA: Admiralty, 101/132; and Bryson, *Report on the Climate and Principal Diseases*, 232.

54. Dornin to Isaac Tousey. USS San Jacinto, At Sea. August 9, 1860. HL: HM30206. Thomas Aloysius Dornin. Letterbook, May 15, 1860–Sept. 16, 1861.

55. Ship Asseiceira. March 31, 1841. AHI: Coleçoes Especiais. Comissão Mista. Brasil—Grã Bretanha (Tráfico de negros). Lata 02, Maço 02, Pasta 01.

56. Watt, "The Health of Seamen," 73.

57. Entry of March 24/25, 1849. AHM: Brigue Mondego/1. Diário Naútico (1849).

58. In Cuba, for example, the use of vinegar was recommended during the months of June, July, and August alongside "the fumigation of Guyton Morveau," in order to cover the smell of urine resulting from sick slaves; Chateausaulin, *El vademecum de los hacendados cubanos*, 46–47.

59. Bryson, *Report on the Climate and Principal Diseases*, 225.

60. Ibid.

61. Ibid., 119; and Clarke, *Sierra Leone*, 72.

62. Boyle, *A Practical Medico-Historical Account*, 11–12.

63. Bethell, "The Mixed Commission," 81–82; Brown, "Fernando Po"; and Lynn, "Britain's West African Policy." On Spain's control over Fernando Po see Emily Berquist Soulé, "From Africa to the Ocean Sea: Atlantic Slavery in the Origins of the Spanish Empire," *Atlantic Studies* 15, no. 1 (2018): 16–39.

64. Joaquim Bento de Fonseca to ?. Quartel, May 19, 1828. ANTT: Documentos de Negócios Estrangeiros. Arquivo Central. Commissões Mistas. Caixa 224. Sierra Leone Papers.

65. Ibid. See also "Coast of Africa," *The Observer*, December 13, 1829, 2.

66. Proposals to situate the British colonial government headquarters at Fernando Po were discussed in years to come, notably in the mid-1830s, when MacGregor Laird and R. A. K. Oldfield recommended it as the place with the best geo-

graphical position to support the activities of the Royal Navy; Laird and Oldfield, *Narrative of an Expedition into the Interior*, 391.

67. Clarke, "Short Notes on the Prevailing Diseases," 64.

68. Couling, *History of the temperance movement.*

69. Carpenter, *The Physiology of Temperance*, 102, 148–49.

70. Clarke, "Short Notes on the Prevailing Diseases," 76.

71. Leonard, *Records of a Voyage to the Western Coast of Africa*, 76; Carpenter, *The Physiology of Temperance*, 148–49.

72. Bryson, *Report on the Climate and Principal Diseases*, 209.

73. A. Nicholl to the Governor. Sierra Leone, January 24, 1820. SLPA: Governor Despatches, 1818–22.

74. Augustus P. Arkwright to his mother. HMS Pantaloon, Sierra Leone, January 22, 1842. DRO: D5991/10/71.

75. Response of William Ferguson. Sierra Leone, April 24, 1826. Sierra Leone Commissions of Enquiry. Vol. 2, Appendixes B and C. TNA: Colonial Office, 267/92.

76. Candler and Wilson were specifically referring to the behavior of British sailors; Candler and Burgess, *Narrative of a Recent Visit to Brazil*, 81.

77. See, for example, Philalethes and Alfaro, *Yankee Travels*, 206; and Howe, *A Trip to Cuba*, 78.

78. Reece, *Medical Guide for Tropical Climates*, 206.

79. Canney, *Africa Squadron*, 124–25.

80. H. J. Ricketts to C. L. F. Haenzel. Government House, Freetown, April 10, 1829. HCPP: Papers Relating to the Colony of Sierra Leone. Ordered by The House of Commons, to be printed, February 17, 1830, 46.

81. Katherine Paugh has noted that since the seventeenth and eighteenth centuries European medical authorities had believed that "the great pox," a generic term to refer to diseases such as yaws and syphilis, had "its origins in the sexual excesses of tropical men and women"; Paugh, "Yaws, Syphilis, Sexuality," 226.

82. Boyle, *A Practical Medico-Historical Account*, 291.

83. John Young to Governor Middlemore. Custom House, St. Helena, June 11, 1840. SHGA: Colonial Secretary's Letters 9, 1841–42.

84. Mayer, *Captain Canot*, 81, 187 (for Ormond); and 263 (for De Souza). For a description of Pedro Blanco's native wives' dwellings see Hall, "Abolition of the Slave Trade of Gallinas," 34. For a further discussion of De Souza's "wives" and other family, see Ana Lucía Araujo, *Public Memory of Slavery: Victims and Perpetrators in the South Atlantic* (Amherst, NY: Cambria, 2010), 302–4.

85. Puga to John Gonzalez (on his ship). Gallinas, [1838]. TNA: Foreign Office, 315/82.

86. J. Jacintho J. Jor. to Alvaro Correia de Morais (at Onim). Bahia, December 16, 1844. TNA: Foreign Office, 315/53.

87. Fernández de Madrid, "Memoria sobre la disentería," 394.

88. Deposition of Nambey. Montego Bay, July 4, 1838. See Barcia, "White Cannibals, Enslaved Africans." For the *Jesús María* case see "Horrors of the Slave Trade," *The Friend: A Religious and Literary Journal* 16, no. 50 (1843): 395.

89. The case can be found in TNA: Foreign Office 84/383 and 313/62. See also Dalleo, "Africans in the Caribbean"; Dorsey, *Slave Trade in the Age of Abolition,* 136–46; and Van Norman, "The Process of Cultural Change."

90. W. H. Macaulay and R. Doherty to Lord Palmerston. Sierra Leone, October 31, 1838. HCPP: Correspondence with British Commissioners at Sierra Leone, Havana, Rio de Janeiro and Surinam on Slave Trade, 1838–39 (Class A, Further Series), 1.

91. Some of these same men, including two clerks and HMS *Bonetta*'s assistant surgeon, Charles Jolley, were reported dead only a few days after the drawing was made. See William Winniett to Chard. [HMS *Viper*], Off Bonny, April 2, [1838]. OUWL: Thomas Fowell Buxton Papers. Sections A–B. Mss. British Empire s. 444 (27).

92. Nelson, "Slavery, Race, and Conspiracy."

93. See, for example, Reece, *Medical Guide for Tropical Climates;* Bryson, *Report on the Climate and Principal Diseases;* Clarke, *Sierra Leone;* and McWilliam, *Medical History of the Expedition to the Niger.*

94. Reece, *Medical Guide for Tropical Climates,* 205–9.

95. McWilliam, *Medical History of the Expedition to the Niger,* 16–23.

96. Robert Clarke to R. D. Ross, Acting Colonial Secretary. Colonial Hospital, Cape Coast, May 10, 1859. TNA: Colonial Office, 100/14.

97. Informação sobre as visitas do corpo de saúde nos navios que entram no porto de Rio de Janeiro. By the Barão da Saúde (Francisco Manuel de Paula). Rio de Janeiro, January 27, 1828. ANRJ: Códice 1091, vol. 1, fol. 18. Cf. Rodrigues, *De Costa a Costa,* 292.

98. Among those were the vessels *Maria da Gloria* in 1834 (TNA: Foreign Office, 315/66); *Segunda Iberia* in 1836 (TNA: Foreign Office, 315/78); *Orozimbo* in 1840 (TNA: Foreign Office, 315/50); and *Izabel* in 1851 (TNA: Foreign Office, 315/96).

99. Description of a Packet found on board the "Vivo." Batua, December 26, 1844. HCPP: Correspondence with British Coms. at Sierra Leone, Havana, Cape of Good Hope, Jamaica, Loanda, and Cape Verd Islands; Reports from British Vice-Admiralty Courts and Naval Officers on Slave Trade, 1845 (Class A), 231.

100. See, for example, the case of the brig *Destemida,* seized and taken to Sierra
     Leone in 1839. Report of the case of the brig "Destemida," Manoel Francisco
     Pinto, captain of the Portuguese flag. Sierra Leone, November 30, 1839.
     HCPP: Correspondence with British Coms. at Sierra Leone, Havana, Rio de
     Janeiro and Surinam on Slave Trade, 1840 (Class A), 257.
101. Rodrigues, *De Costa a Costa,* 174.
102. Ibid.
103. See, for example, Harrison, "Quarantine, Pilgrimage, and Colonial Trade";
     Birsen Bulmus, *Plague, Quarantines, and Geopolitics;* Tognotti, "Lessons from
     the History of Quarantine"; Longhurst, "Quarantine Matters"; and Bashford,
     Quarantine.
104. Bashford, "Maritime Quarantine," 2, 6.
105. Clarke, *Sierra Leone,* 72–73; Thomas Cole to John Doherty. Liberated Afri-
     can Department, September 12, 1829. SLPA: Liberated African Department
     Letterbook, 1828–30; Hamilton to Canning. Sierra Leone, October 12, 1826.
     TNA: Foreign Office, 84/49 (ii). For the smallpox hospital at Wilberforce see
     the records concerning the Spanish schooner *Iberia.* January 27, 1826. SLPA:
     Liberated African Department. Statement of Disposals, 1821–33.
106. See the numerous notices sent by Captain General Marquis of Someruelos
     from 1802 onward. ANC: Miscelánea de Libros, 6756. See also "Estados y ac-
     tuaciones sobre fiebre amarilla y parte mensual sanitario, desde 18 Diciembre
     de 1837 hasta 31 de Diciembre de 1858." ANC: Junta Superior de Sanidad, 13/3.
107. See also Duarte, *Ensaio sobre a hygiene da escravatura no Brasil,* 4–5; and
     Mattos, "Do que eles padeciam . . .," 71–73.
108. Bashford, "Maritime Quarantine," 5.
109. Zayas, Carrillo, Cascales y Ariza and Chacón y Calvo to the Count of Ricafort.
     Havana, April 9, 1833. ANC: Asuntos Políticos, 35/47. Ricafort eventually
     heeded their call and ordered even stricter quarantine regulations.
110. José María Govín and Miguel Antonio Madruga to the Captain General.
     Matanzas, November 2, 1820. ANC: Gobierno Superior Civil, 870/29386.
111. Captain General Miguel Tacón to the Mixed Commissioners. Havana, March
     7, 1836. HCPP: Correspondence with British Coms. at Sierra Leone, Havana,
     Rio de Janeiro and Surinam on Slave Trade, 1836 (Class A), 141–42.
112. Angel José Cowley and Antonio Maria de la Torre to the Captain General.
     Havana, March 6, 1836. Antonio Ursaiz and Antonio Maria de la Torre to the
     Captain General. Office of the Captain of the Port, Havana, March 6, 1836.
     Ibid., 141–42.
113. McHenry to Lord Stanley. St. Helena, April 13, 1843. SHGA: Colonial Secre-
     tary's Letters, 14 (1843).

114. Burton, *Wanderings in West Africa,* 1: 18.

115. Graden, *Disease, Resistance, and Lies,* 70–74.

116. López Denis, "Cuerpos y prácticas"; and Beldarraín Chaple, "Las epidemias y su enfrentamiento." See also ANC: Junta Superior de Sanidad, Book 14, sessions of October 16, 1831, and December 17, 1831.

117. Hamilton to Canning. Sierra Leone, October 12, 1826. TNA: Foreign Office, 84/49 (ii).

118. Colonial Surgeon (Ferguson) to Colonial Secretary (J. Reffell). Collector's Office, May 24, 1826. Ibid.

119. [Bel], "Mémoire sur l'épidémie," 206.

120. Burton, *Wanderings in West Africa,* 1: 18.

121. William Barry to the Acting Governor. Freetown, April 20, 1826. SLPA: Liberated African Department Letterbook, 1820–26, vol. 1.

122. George McDonald to W. N. Aitkin. Secretary's Office. Sierra Leone, November 11, 1844. SLPA: Colonial Secretary's Letterbook. November 11, 1844–September 29, 1845.

123. Ouseley, *Notes on the Slave-Trade,* 25–26.

124. W. S. Macleay and Edward W. H. Schenley to Palmerston. Havana, December 29, 1835. HCPP: Correspondence with British Coms. at Sierra Leone, Havana, Rio de Janeiro and Surinam on Slave Trade: 1835 (Class A), 200–201; and Macleay and Schenley to Palmerston. Havana, December 31, 1835. TNA: Foreign Office 84/172.

125. Hamilton to Canning. Sierra Leone, October 12, 1826. TNA: Foreign Office, 84/49 (ii); and M[ichael]. L. Melville and James Hook to Lord Aberdeen. Sierra Leone, November 15, 1844. TNA: Foreign Office, 84/507B.

126. Cardoso to the Baron of Lazarim. Luanda, aboard the Mondego, July 15, 1844. AHM: Documentação Avulsa, Caixa 471–71, Brigue Mondego.

127. Cardoso to the Baron of Lazarim. Luanda, aboard the Mondego, July 13, 1849. Ibid.

128. See for example the story of a young African boy suffering from smallpox, who was murdered by Theodore Canot during the Atlantic crossing, in order to prevent the spread of the diseases among slaves and crew. Mayer, *Captain Canot,* 276–80.

Chapter 2. The Blood of Thousands

1. "Transfers of slaves upon the death of the Captain and Surgeon (Le Jeune Louis) At sea 4 degrees latitude South, 13 degrees longitude West." HL: French

Clandestine Slave Trade Collection, HM45994. For a more in-depth discussion of this case see Fohlen, "Une expédition négrière nantaise."

2. Angelucci to the Knights of San Juan de Dios. Havana, July 23, 1825. HL: French Clandestine Slave Trade Collection, HM44028.

3. Miscellaneous records of expenditures relating to the "Jeune Louis" at Havana. Ibid.

4. Luciano Belloch to Vilardaga. Ouidah, July 1, 1830. TNA: Foreign Office, 315/75. He was probably referring here to Benito Torrent and Joaquín Bergallo, two well-known slave ship captains of the late 1820s.

5. R. B. Estrada, *Geografía. Relación de un viaje a las islas de cabo Verde, y algunos puntos del y Río Pongo.* Biblioteca Nacional de Cuba: CM Bachiller: (1833/4). Cf. Zeuske, *Amistad,* 152.

6. Estrada, *Geografía.*

7. Ibid.

8. Ysabel Klem to her son Ysidro Powell. Cárdenas, August 14 and 30, 1830. TNA: Foreign Office, 315/66.

9. Contract signed on November 17, 1819 in Santiago de Cuba by Mariano Carbó, captain of the schooner Gaceta and the ship owners, Rafael Alcón, Cosme Giménes, and Francisco Sánchez. TNA: Foreign Office, 315/71.

10. Lombillo to Ozquiano. Havana, February 7, 1818. TNA: Foreign Office, 315/56. As we have seen, during the Middle Passage slave traders could resort to murdering slaves who were suspected to be a threat to the rest on board. Mayer, *Captain Canot,* 276–80.

11. Lombillo to Ozquiano. Havana, February 7, 1818. TNA: Foreign Office, 315/56.

12. Teixeira to Abranxes. Benguela, February 24, 1839. "Embarcação: Especulador. 1839." AHI: Coleções Especiais. 33. Comissões Mistas (Tráfico de Negros). Brasil—Grã Bretanha. Lata 14, Maço 3, Pasta 1. For a discussion on fabricated routes between Benguela, Montevideo, and Mozambique see Ferreira, "The Suppression of the Slave Trade," 318–19.

13. Pedro Martinez and Co. to Jiménez. Havana, September 26, 1838. TNA: Foreign Office, 315/83.

14. Ibid. Slave revolts were a common feature of the post-1820 slave trade. For a well-documented case for this period see "Auto de perguntas feitas ao réu Lauriano, preto de nação Macua"; and "Auto de perguntas feitas ao réu Umpopulha, preto de nação Macua," 1823. APEB: Insurreções de Escravos, 2845. See also Canot's description of an African slave revolt on board the *Estrella;* Mayer, *Captain Canot,* 272–75.

15. Abstract of Evidence in the Case of the "Voladora." Havana, July 1829. TNA: Foreign Office, 84/92.

16. "Criminales seguidos por la aprehensión de una expedición negrera en el Estero de las Brujas, jurisdicción de Trinidad, 1854." ANC: Miscelánea de Expedientes, 781/L.

17. See, for example, Mayer, *Captain Canot,* 276.

18. Deposition of José Joaquim de Moraes. Anglo-Portuguese Mixed Commission Court, Rio de Janeiro. Session of July 13, 1821. ANRJ: Libro de Protocolos das Conferencias da Comissão Mixta sobre o Tráfico da Escravatura. Junta do Comércio. Códice 184, Vol. 2.

19. "Matrícula da Equipagem do Brique Bom Caminho, que segue viagem para Molembo (1823)" TNA: Foreign Office, 315/62; and "Matrícula da Equipagem da Escuna Bella Eliza que segue viagem para Molembo (1824)" TNA: Foreign Office, 315/63.

20. On sangradores see, for example, Pimenta, "Entre sangradores e doutores"; and Santana and Oliveira dos Santos, "Sangradores Africanos."

21. Pimenta, "Entre sangradores e doutores," 94.

22. On this issue, see, for example, Rodrigues, *De Costa a Costa,* 276–77.

23. Zeuske, "Cosmopólitas del Atlántico esclavista."

24. Matson, *Remarks on the Slave Trade,* 46–47. See also Forçade to François Barraillier. Havana, May 15, 1839. HCPP: 1841 Session 1 [330] Correspondence with the British commissioners at Sierra Leone, the Havana, Rio de Janeiro, and Surinam, relating to the slave trade. May 11–December 31, 1840, inclusive (Class A), 118.

25. Testimonies of William Laurenson and William Henry Christie. Rio de Janeiro, July 22 and 23, 1847. SML: Despatches from United States Consuls in Rio de Janeiro, 1811–1906. Vols. 11 and 12. September 1, 1845–December 25, 1848.

26. Puga to Domingo Novo (at the Wharf of Horses in Havana). [Gallinas], n/d, 1838. TNA: Foreign Office, 315/82.

27. Testimony of Joseph Alvares Cunha. Rio de Janeiro, July 20, 1847. SML: Despatches from United States Consuls in Rio de Janeiro, 1811–1906. Vols. 11 and 12. September 1, 1845–December 25, 1848.

28. Testimony of William Laurenson. Rio de Janeiro, July 23, 1847. SML: Despatches from United States Consuls in Rio de Janeiro, 1811–1906. Vols. 11 and 12. September 1, 1845–December 25, 1848.

29. Ibid.

30. Joaquim Antonio Lima to Joaquim Pereira de Mendonça. Loanda, February 3, 1842. "Embarcação: Aracaty. 1842." AHI: Coleções Especiais, 53. Comissões Mistas (Tráfico de Negros). Brasil—Grã Bretanha. Lata 2, Maço 1, Pasta 1.

31. Letter from the Vigilante's crew to [Francisco Romagoza?], n/d, 1838. TNA: Foreign Office, 315/84.

32. Depositions of Antonio Congo and Dominga Conga. Remedios, n/d, 1858. ANC: Miscelánea de Expedientes, 3830/At.

33. Ibid.

34. See, among others found in the same document, the testimonies of Mary, or Manu, and Sadea, or Sarah. Lucea, July 18, 1838. HCPP: 1839 (157) *Slave Trade. Copy of the report of Hall Pringle and Alexander Campbell, Esquires, associate justices of the peace, relatives to certain atrocities of slave trades*, 2, 3.

35. Ibid.

36. Barnard, *A Three Years' Cruize.*

37. In February 1846, Barnard was again reassigned to serve on board HMS *Cleopatra.* O'Byrne, *Naval Biographical Dictionary*, 48.

38. Barnard, *A Three Years' Cruize*, 19.

39. Ibid., 154.

40. Ibid., 137.

41. Ibid., 138.

42. See, for example, Soumonni, "Lacustrine Villages in South Benin."

43. Law, *Ouidah,* 137. See also Sparks, *Where the Negroes are Masters.*

44. See, for example, Fett, *Recaptured Africans,* 54, 58, 72; Ferreira, "Measuring Short- and Long-Term Impacts," 228–29; Candido, *An African Slaving Port,* 169–70; and Domingues da Silva, *The Atlantic Slave Trade.*

45. Ouseley, *Notes on the Slave-Trade,* 50.

46. Boubacar Barry has described the practice by slave dealers at Rio Pongo from the 1820s, of using their slaves to grow coffee during the rainy seasons, only to send them away into the transatlantic slave trade during the following dry seasons; Barry, *Senegambia and the Atlantic Slave Trade,* 133–35.

47. Mouser, "The Baltimore/Pongo Connection"; Mouser, "A History of the Rio Pongo"; and Kelly and Fall, "Employing Archaeology." Something very similar was also going on along the Angolan coast during this period. See Ferreira, *Dos Sertões ao Atlântico,* 107–8.

48. Deposition of Sulimana, a slave on board the Rosalia. [Freetown], January 21, 1822. TNA: Foreign Office, 315/72.

49. Deposition of Jumo. [Freetown], January 21, 1822. Ibid.

50. Von Zütphen, *Tagebuch einer Reise,* 34.

51. Testimonies of Zebina H. Small Jr., and Ebenezer B. Burgess. On board the *Sea Eagle* at Rio de Janeiro, November 27 and 28, 1844. SML: Despatches from United States Consuls in Rio de Janeiro, 1811–1906, Vol. 8. January 3, 1845–March 26, 1845.

52. [Fawkner], *Narrative,* 117.

53. Melville and Hook to the Earl of Aberdeen. Sierra Leone, December 31, 1844. Correspondence with British Coms. at Sierra Leone, Havana, Cape of Good Hope, Jamaica, Loanda, and Cape Verd Islands; Reports from British Vice-Admiralty Courts and Naval Officers on Slave Trade: 1845 (Class A), 5–6. For a discussion on the effects of waiting times in barracoons along the coast, especially in the last years of the illegal slave trade see Harris, "Yankee 'Blackbirding,' " 129–30.

54. Rapport sur l'etat actuel de la traite des noirs by Commandant Auguste Baudin. Gorée, April 3, 1845. ANOM: Généralités, 166/1341.

55. Report of the Case of the Portuguese Brig "Emprendedor," Francisco G. Veiga, Master. Sierra Leone, December 11, 1838. HCPP: Correspondence with British Coms. at Sierra Leone, Havana, Rio de Janeiro and Surinam on Slave Trade: 1839–40 (Class A), 95.

56. Ibid.

57. Mayer, *Captain Canot,* 402–4.

58. Commodore Wilmot to the Sec. of the Admiralty. HMS Rattlesnake, at Ascension, December 1, 1864. HCCP: Correspondence with British Coms. at Sierra Leone, Havana, Cape of Good Hope and Loanda; Reports from British Naval Forces on Slave Trade: 1864 (Class A), 152.

59. Ibid.

60. Depositions of Sulimana and Jumo. [Freetown], January 21, 1822. TNA: Foreign Office, 315/72.

61. Baudin to the Ministre de la Marine et des Colonies. Gorée docks, November 12, 1844. ANOM: Généralités, 166/1341.

62. Estrada, *Geografía.*

63. Ibid.

64. Barcia, "Fully Capable of Any Iniquity," 316–17.

65. His death was recorded by British missionary Thomas Birch Freeman in his personal journal. See Freeman, *Journal of Various Visits,* 248.

66. Zangroniz to Palau. [Ouidah], August 13, [1836]. TNA: Foreign Office, 315/68.

67. [Jordi] to González Carbajal. Little Bassam, December 15, 1828. TNA: Foreign Office, 315/44.

68. [Jordi] to González Carbajal. Little Bassam, November 23, 1828. Ibid.

69. Turnbull, *Travels in the West,* 60–61.

70. Ibid.

71. "Testimonio de las diligencias formadas por la aprehensión de una expedición de bozales." ANC: Miscelánea de Expedientes, 564/A.

72. Macleay and McKenzie to Lord Palmerston. Havana, September 12, 1833; and Extract from a letter from Mr. Macleay dated Havana, October 3, 1833. TNA: Foreign Office, 84/137.

73. "Insurrección de los esclavos del cafetal Salvador." ANC: Miscelánea de Expedientes, 540/B.

74. Macleay and McKenzie to Lord Palmerston. Havana, September 12, 1833; and Extract from a letter from Mr. Macleay dated Havana, October 3, 1833. TNA: Foreign Office, 84/137.

75. Ibid.

76. Tudor, *Narrative of a Tour in North America*, 2: 131.

77. Madden to Schenley. Havana, September 23, 1836. TNA: Foreign Office, 84/195.

78. Schenley and Madden to the Captain General. Havana, June 16, 1837. TNA: Foreign Office, 84/216.

79. See, for example, Carvalho, *Liberdade;* Silva, "Memórias do tráfico illegal"; Costa, "O Recife nas rotas do Atlântico negro."

80. Testimony of John Parkinson, Esq. HM Consul in Bahia. Bahia, December 10, 1833. HCPP: Correspondence with Foreign Powers, relating to the slave trade, 1834 (Class B), 43.

81. Mattos and Abreu, "Relatório Histórico-Antropológico," 26. See also *Africanos na Santa Casa de Porto Alegre,* 13.

82. "Expediente formado con motivo del apresamiento de un Brick-barca sin bandera, llamado 'Paez,' hecho por el pailebot de guerra 'Cristina' en Los Falcones, jurisdicción de Cárdenas, con 375 bozales." Cárdenas, September 16, 1857. ANC: Asuntos Políticos, 223/7.

83. Testimonies of seamen John Fairburn and James Gillespie. Rio de Janeiro, September 12, 1844. SML: Despatches from United States Consuls in Rio de Janeiro, 1811–1906, Vol. 8. January 3, 1845–March 26, 1845.

84. For the strategies developed by slave traders to avoid capture during the illegal period see Pérez Morales, "Tricks of the Slave Trade"; and Barcia and Kesidou, "Innovation and Entrepreneurship."

85. Belloch to Nocetti. Ouidah, June 21, 1830. TNA: Foreign Office, 315/75.

86. Belloch to Nocetti. Ouidah, June 23, 1830. Ibid.

87. Belloch to Nocetti. Ouidah, June 27, 1830. Ibid.

88. Belloch to Vilardaga. Ouidah, July 1, 1830. Ibid.

89. Calveras to Nocetti. Ouidah, July 7, 1830; and Belloch to Nocetti. Ouidah, July 7, 1830. Ibid.

90. Calveras to Nocetti. Ouidah, August 3, 1830. Ibid.

91. Belloch to Nocetti. Ouidah, August 6, 1830. Ibid.

92. Macleay to the Earl of Aberdeen. Havana, September 2, 1828 and December 15, 1828. TNA: Foreign Office, 84/81.

93. Francisco Jozé Pires de Carvalho (Cirúrgico Maior da Capitanía de Moçambique) to the Governor of Moçambique [Mozambique, May 6, 1819]. AHU: Moçambique. Caixa 162, No. 88 (162/88), 1819.

94. Ibid.

95. "Do Depósito Geral de Medicamentos do Exército. Se Remete para a Ilha de S. Thomé e Principe os Medicamentos Contentos nesta Relacão." AHSTP: Núcleo de S. Tomé, Arquivo da Secretaría-Geral do Governo, Série A (1802–1923), Maço 5: Oficios e portarias da Metrópole (1835), fols. 10–11v.

96. Owen, *Narrative of Voyages*, 1: 296.

97. Ibid.

98. List of medicines on board the Especulador. AHI: "Embarcação: Especulador. 1839." Coleções Especiais. 33. Comissões Mistas (Tráfico de Negros). Brasil—Grã Bretanha. Lata 14, Maço 3, Pasta 1.

99. Método curativo: Viruela. TNA: Foreign Office, 316/76.

100. Ibid.

101. Cloruro de Sosa. Ibid.

102. Ibid.

103. Ibid.

104. "Recetta per lusegetto negro." TNA: Foreign Office, 315/56.

105. "El rob antisifilitico de Laffeteur." Ibid. See also Androutsos, Diamantis, and Vladimiros, "Le 'Rob de Laffecteur.' "

106. Ibid.

107. "Cases in which the contents of this chest must be used." TNA: Foreign Office, 315/89.

108. Ibid. On the Leroy's purgative elixir see Ramsey, "Academic Medicine and Medical Industrialism," esp. 48–51.

109. "Cases in which the contents of this chest must be used." TNA: Foreign Office, 315/89.

110. Ibid.

111. Lefer Robaud to the Duke of San Fernando. Sierra Leone, February 1820. AHN: Estado, 8030/45.

Chapter 3. Cruising for Slaves and Boating Up Rivers

Epigraph. Quoted in Gilliland, *Voyage to the Thousand Cares*, 25.

1. George McLaren's Naval Journals. Port Royal, July 31, 1835. CUMC: MS Add.9528/2.

2. Ibid.

3. Ibid. Havana, January 25, 1836.

4. Ibid. Off Grenada, October 6, 1836.

5. Ibid. Havana, January 10, 1837.

6. See Bethell, "The Mixed Commission"; Martinez-Fernandez, "The Havana Anglo-Spanish Mixed Commission"; Shaikh, "Judicial Diplomacy"; Martinez, *Slave Trade;* and Nelson, "Liberated Africans in the Atlantic World." See also Helfman, "The Court of Vice Admiralty"; and Graden, "Interpreters, Translators, and the Spoken Word."

7. For a short time in the mid-1830s a Brazilian anti-slave trade squadron had some success capturing slave vessels. See Bethell, *The Abolition of the Brazilian Slave Trade,* 177. See also Huzzey, *Freedom Burning;* Scanlan, *Freedom's Debtors;* and Rodrigues, " 'In This Trade, No Places Are Held'. "

8. Canney, *Africa Squadron,* viii.

9. Ibid., 15–28. See also Howarth, *To Shining Sea,* esp. parts II and III; and Head, *Privateers of the Americas.*

10. To date, the most comprehensive study of the French campaign to bring the slave trade to an end is Serge Daget, *La répression de la traite des Noirs.*

11. Gregory and Fitzgerald to the Marquis of Londonderry. Sierra Leone, April 30, 1842. HCPP: Correspondence with British Coms. at Sierra Leone, Havana, Rio de Janeiro and Surinam on Slave Trade: 1822–23 (Class B), 1. Unfortunately, other than Daget's important book, not much has been written about the activities of the French Anti-Slave Trade Squadron during the 1820s and 1830s.

12. Le Capitain de frigate, Commandant la Station extérioure d'Afrique to [Le Ministre de la Marine et des Colonies]. Corvette La Diane, at Gorée, April 1, 1822. ANOM: Généralités. 166/1342.

13. French Consul in Havana to Le Ministre de la Marine et des Colonies. Havana, April 10, 1829. ANOM: Généralités. 166/1342.

14. Ibid.

15. For a list of the condemned vessels on French courts during this period see Daget, *Répertoire des Expéditions Négrières Françaises.* For a specific case, that of *L'Hermoine,* condemned in the court of Cayenne after being seized with 123 Africans on board, see Report from the French Naval station on the Coast of Africa. Station Extérieure d'Afrique, February 7, 1827. HCPP: Correspondence with British Coms. at Sierra Leone, Havana, Rio de Janeiro and Surinam on Slave Trade, 1827 (Class A); Correspondence with Foreign Powers on Slave Trade, 1827 (Class B), 279–81.

16. In 1838 British trader Michael Procter complained in a letter to Thomas Fowell Buxton about the fact that British anti-slave trade commanders were "so taken

up with calculations of Prize Money" that they had neglected paying any atten-
tion to British subjects like him, trading along the West African coast. Michael
Procter to [Thomas Fowell Buxton]. Rio Nunez, May 31, 1838. OUWL:
Thomas Fowell Buxton Papers. Sections E-F. Mss. British Empire s. 444 (29).

17. Scanlan, "The Colonial Rebirth of British Anti-Slavery," 1088; see also Scanlan, "The Rewards of Their Exertions."

18. For the capture of the *Butterfly* see United States v. Isaac Morris, 39 U.S. 14 Pet.
464 (1840). For a detailed discussion of both the *Butterfly* and the *Catharine*
cases see Gordan, *This Practice against the Law.*

19. The deployment of this squadron was to a large extent a result of the Webster-
Ashburton treaty of 1842. The most extensive study on this treaty is Jones, *To
the Webster-Ashburton Treaty.* See also Jones, "The Influence of Slavery on the
Webster-Ashburton Negotiations"; and Marques, *The United States and the
Transatlantic Slave Trade,* 137.

20. Cole and Macaulay to Palmerston. Sierra Leone, January 5, 1835. HCPP: Correspondence with British Coms. at Sierra Leone, Havana, Rio de Janeiro and
Surinam on Slave Trade: 1835 (Class A), 2.

21. Palmerston to Viscount Granville. Foreign Office, 15 July 1831; and Granville to
Palmerston. Paris, July 18, 1831. HCPP: Correspondence with British Coms. at
Sierra Leone, Havana, Rio de Janeiro and Surinam, and with Foreign Powers
on Slave Trade, 1831 (Class A & B), 183–84.

22. Enclosure 9 in No. 187. Divisions and Stations of the French Squadron employed in the Suppression of the Slave Trade on the West Coast of Africa, on
April 30, 1846. HCPP: Correspondence with British Coms. at Sierra Leone,
Havana, Cape of Good Hope, Jamaica, Loanda, and Cape Verde Islands; Reports from British Vice-Admiralty Courts and Naval Officers on Slave Trade,
1846 (Class A), 337.

23. W. H. Macaulay to Lord Aberdeen. Cape Verde Islands, May 25, 1846. Ibid.,
326.

24. See, for example, Admiral Massien [de Clerval] to the Ministre de Marine. Rio de
Janeiro, December 25, 1841. HCPP: Correspondence with British Coms. at Sierra
Leone, Havana, Rio de Janeiro and Surinam on Slave Trade: 1835 (Class A), 5.

25. Bouët-Willaumez was in command of the West African squadron between 1844
and 1845, and then again between 1848 and 1850. Baudin also had two spells
in charge, first in 1848, and then between 1851 and 1854. The former also left
a written account of his experiences fighting the slave trade. See Bouët-
Willaumez, *Commerce et Traite.*

26. Baudin went as far as Cabinda in this scouting mission. While visiting the Upper Guinea coast he found Pedro Blanco's former factory at Joury and Theo-

dore Canot's abandoned plantations at Cape Mount. See Rapport sur l'état actuel de la traite des noirs. Gorée, April 3, 1845. ANOM: Généralités, 166/1341. See also Baudin to the Ministre de la Marine et des Colonies. Gorée docks, November 12, 1844. Ibid.

27. De Monleón to the Baron de Mackau. Brig La Zèbre, Sierra Leone, February 19, 1845. Ibid. During this assignment de Monleón attacked and destroyed the slave factory of Andrés Jiménez at Gallinas.

28. *L'Australie* had been taking supplies at Luanda at least from 1847. AHM: Livro de Registo de Quartos (1847–48), Brigue Mondego/4, 1199; fol. 84.

29. Edmund Gabriel and G. Brand to Lord Aberdeen. Luanda, June 7, 1846. HCPP: Correspondence with British Coms. at Sierra Leone, Havana, Cape of Good Hope, Jamaica, Loanda, and Cape Verde Islands; Reports from British Vice-Admiralty Courts and Naval Officers on Slave Trade, 1846 (Class A), 309.

30. Massinon, "L'enterprise du Rio-Nunez"; Braithwaite, "The Rio Nuñez Affair"; and Braithwaite, *Palmerston and Africa.*

31. George Jackson and Edmund Gabriel to Palmerston. Luanda, February 18, 1847. HCPP: Correspondence with British Coms. at Sierra Leone, Havana, Cape of Good Hope, Jamaica, Loanda, and Cape Verde Islands; Reports from British Vice-Admiralty Courts and Naval Officers on Slave Trade: 1847–March 1848 (Class A), 154; and Her Majesty's Commissioners to Palmerston. Luanda, February 5, 1850. HCPP: Correspondence with British Coms. at Sierra Leone, Havana, Cape of Good Hope, Jamaica, Loanda, and Cape Verde Islands; Reports from British Vice-Admiralty Courts and Naval Officers on Slave Trade, 1850–51 (Class A), 59. See also Candido, *An African Slaving Port,* 151–52, 160–70.

32. George Jackson to Palmerston. Luanda, January 26, 1851. HCPP: Correspondence with British Coms. at Sierra Leone, Havana, Cape of Good Hope, Jamaica, Loanda, and Cape Verde Islands; Reports from British Vice-Admiralty Courts and Naval Officers on Slave Trade: April 1851–March 1852 (Class A), 119.

33. Ferreira, *The Costs of Freedom,* especially chapters 4 and 5.

34. Livro de Registro de Quartos (1848). AHM: Brigue Mondego/4; fol. 1199.

35. Commodore Hotham to the Secretary of the Admiralty. Penelope, Sierra Leone, February 12, 1849. HCPP: Correspondence with British Ministers and Agents in Foreign Countries, and with Foreign Ministers in England, on Slave Trade, 1849–50 (Class B), 216.

36. Commodore Fanshawe to the Secretary of the Admiralty. Centaur, at sea, April 29, 1851. HCPP: Correspondence with British Coms. at Sierra Leone, Havana, Cape of Good Hope, Jamaica, Loanda, and Cape Verde Islands; Reports from

British Vice-Admiralty Courts and Naval Officers on Slave Trade: April 1851–March 1852 (Class A), 230.

37. Commodore Hotham to the Secretary of the Admiralty. Penelope, Sierra Leone, February 12, 1849. HCPP: Correspondence with British Ministers and Agents in Foreign Countries, and with Foreign Ministers in England, on Slave Trade, 1849–50 (Class B), 216–67.

38. For example, in 1845 HMS *Lily* stopped and searched the American barque *Madonna,* provoking a strong reaction from the U.S. government. In a similar incident, in 1860 HMS *Falcon* detained the American vessel *Jehossee,* leading to a number of threatening letters between U.S. and British naval officers. See Canney, *Africa Squadron,* 79; and William Inman to Captain R. W. Courtenay. USS Constellation, St. Paul of Luanda, February 4, 1860; Courtenay to Inman. Archer, February 9, 1860; and Inman to Courtenay. Constellation, St. Paul of Luanda, February 11, 1860. HCPP: Correspondence with British Coms. at Sierra Leone, Havana, Cape of Good Hope and Loanda; Reports from British Naval Forces on Slave Trade, April 1860–March 1861 (Class A), 64–65.

39. Lord Lyons to Seward. Washington DC, August 30, 1861; and Seward to Lord Lyons. Washington DC, December 10, 1861. HCPP: Correspondence with British Ministers and Agents in Foreign Countries, and with Foreign Ministers in England, on Slave Trade, 1861 (Class B), 164, 171.

40. Canney, *Africa Squadron,* 233–34; and Harris, "Yankee 'Blackbirding.' "

41. Miguel Tacón to ?. Barcelona, June 27, 1844. AHN: Estado, 8035, no. 4.

42. Charles Pennell to Canning. Bahia, June 1, 1827. TNA: Foreign Office, 84/287. See also the report by Joaquim de Paula Guedes Alcoforado. "Relatorio Feito Pelo Alcoforado sobre o trafico, 1831–1853." ANRJ: Ministério da Justiça, IJ6-525; and Marques, "The Contraband Slave Trade to Brazil."

43. Filho, *O negro na Bahia,* 88.

44. Bethell, *The Abolition of the Brazilian Slave Trade,* 180–241; Parron, *A política da escravidão no Império do Brasil,* 159–60.

45. Marques, *The Sounds of Silence,* 123–26.

46. In 1850 Henry Huntley commented on life aboard an anti–slave trade patrol: "The mids [midshipmen] speculated upon their respective prospects of becoming prize masters. The commander and the assistant surgeon, paced the deck, calculating their chances of prize-money and promotion"; Huntley, *Seven Years Service,* 1: 97.

47. Owen, *Narrative of Voyages,* 1: 151.

48. Ibid.

49. Leonard, *Records of a Voyage to the Western Coast of Africa,* 40.

50. Ibid., 16.

51. Clemente Joaquim d'Abranches Bisarro (surgeon). Aboard Brig Audaz, February 1, 1841. AHM: Documentação Avulsa, Caixa 468-2, Brigue Audaz (1820–53).
52. Journals of James Nicholas Dick, British naval surgeon, and James Douglas Dick, naval officer, 1853–98. BAC: Rare Books and Manuscripts, DA88.1.D53.
53. Barcia, *West African Warfare in Bahia,* 73–79.
54. Pérez Morales, "Tricks of the Slave Trade"; and Barcia and Kesidou, "Innovation and Entrepreneurship."
55. Dunlop to Fanny Dunlop. HMS Alert, Sierra Leone, October 17, 1849. NMM: MS87/002. Letters of Hugh Dunlop, 1842–61.
56. Dunlop to Fanny. HMS Alert, Sierra Leone, January 14, 1850. Ibid. On the Kroomen and their relationship with anti–slave trade squadrons in West Africa see Burroughs, "The True Sailors of Western Africa."
57. "Attack on Medina, Sierra Leone River," *Illustrated London News,* May 14, 1853, 368.
58. Mr. Thornton to Commander Need. Crawford Island, August 11, 1853. NMM: MS65/134. Art/10 Album.
59. Journals of James Nicholas Dick, British naval surgeon, and James Douglas Dick, naval officer, 1853–98. BAC: Rare Books and Manuscripts. DA88.1.D53.
60. Ibid.
61. Arkwright to his Grandfather. HMS Prompt, becalmed off Sierra Leone, November 7, 1842. DRO: D5991/10/74.
62. Gilliland, *Voyage to the Thousand Cares,* 32.
63. Journal kept by Ernest de Cornulier. French Navy, 1822–23. NMM: LOG/F/4.
64. Bryson, *Report on the Climate and Principal Diseases,* 19.
65. Ibid., 132–33.
66. Vicente José dos Santos Moreira Lima to the Major General d'Armada. Brig Audaz, Port of Luanda, April 21, 1839. AHM: Documentação Avulsa, caixa 468-2. Brigue Audaz (1820–53).
67. "Estado actual da Guarniçao do Brigue de Guerra Tejo." Observations by Francisco António Gonçalves Cardoso, February 24, 1840. AHM: Documentação Avulsa, caixa 474-1, Brigue Tejo (1837–40).
68. Cardoso to Vasconcellos Pereira, Major General d'Armada. Luanda, aboard the Tejo, June 30, 1841. AHM: Documentação Avulsa, caixa 474-2. Brigue Tejo (1841–51).
69. Owen, *Narrative of Voyages,* 1: 223–24.
70. "General Intelligence," *National Anti-Slavery Standard,* Monrovia (Thursday, March 18, 1841), 2.
71. Gavin, "Palmerston Policy towards East and West Africa," 138.

72. Trelawney to the Secretary of State for the Colonies. St. Helena, June 11, 1842. TNA: Colonial Office, 247/57.

73. Vowell to Trelawney. St. Helena, June 11, 1842. TNA: Colonial Office, 247/58.

74. Deposition of Henry James Matson. March 28, 1848. HCPP: First report from the Select Committee on Slave Trade, 1847–48, 84.

75. Matson, *Remarks on the Slave Trade,* 39; Foote, *Africa and the American Flag,* 241–42.

76. Baudin to the Ministre de la Marine et des Colonies. Gorée docks, November 12, 1844. ANOM: Généralités, 166/1341.

77. Commodore Hotham to the Secretary of the Admiralty. Penelope, Sierra Leone, February 12, 1849. HCPP: Correspondence with British Ministers and Agents in Foreign Countries, and with Foreign Ministers in England, on Slave Trade, 1849–50 (Class B), 216; and Jackson to Lord Palmerston. Luanda, January 25, 1851. HCPP: Correspondence with British Coms. at Sierra Leone, Havana, Cape of Good Hope, Jamaica, Loanda, and Cape Verd Islands; Reports from British Vice-Admiralty Courts and Naval Officers on Slave Trade: April 1851–March 1852 (Class A), 119. See also Ferreira, "Suppression of the Slave Trade"; and Guizelin, "A abolição do tráfico de escravos no Atlântico Sul."

78. Commodore William Jones to the Lt. Gov. of Sierra Leone. "Penelope," off Gallinas, February 24, 1845. HCPP: Correspondence with the British Commissioners at Sierra Leone, Havana, Rio de Janeiro, Surinam, Cape of Good Hope, Jamaica, Loanda, and Boa Vista relating to the Slave Trade. From January 1 to December 31, 1845 (Class A), 38. Huzzey, *Freedom Burning,* 115–16.

79. Jones to the Lt. Gov. of Sierra Leone. Penelope, Sierra Leone, February 7, 1845. Ibid.

80. Ibid.

81. R. B. Crawford to Rear-Admiral Josceline Percy. HMS Mutini, Pomba Bay, East Coast of Africa, November 25, 1845; Crawford to Pinho. HMS Mutini, Pomba Bay, November 23, 1845; and Pinho to Crawford. Brig Villa Flor, November 23 and 25, 1845. HCPP: Accounts and Papers: Slave Trade. Session January 19–July 23, 1847. Vol. 34, 33–34.

82. "The Slave-Trade in the Mozambique Channel," *Illustrated London News,* January 18, 1851, 44.

83. Leonard, *Records of a Voyage to the Western Coast of Africa,* 259–60; Tinnie, "The Slaving Brig *Henriqueta* and Her Evil Sisters."

84. Pennell to Canning. Bahia, September 20, 1826. HCPP: Correspondence with Foreign Powers on Slave Trade, 1826–27 (Class B), 99. See also Barcia and Kesidou, "Innovation and Entrepreneurship," 542–61.

85. HMS *Hope* had been at sea offering "shelter and comfort" to officers and crews of the West African squadron by staying out at sea, far from the African "unhealthy climate." Extract of a Letter from Commodore Bullen, C. B. to J. W. Croker, Esq.; dated on board H. M. Ship Maidstone, West Bay, Prince's Island, September 15, 1826. HCPP: Papers relating to Slave Trade: Correspondence between Admiralty and Naval Officers on Suppression of Slave Trade, 1825–27, 9–10.

86. Macleay to Aberdeen. Havana, July 3, 1829. HCPP: Correspondence with British Coms. at Sierra Leone, Havana, Rio de Janeiro and Surinam on Slave Trade, 1829 (Class A), 142–43.

87. Ibid.

88. Macleay to Aberdeen. Havana, July 17, 1829. Ibid., 148–49.

89. Examination of Commander William Broughton, Esq. Commander of the H.M. said ship Primrose. HCPP: Correspondence with British Coms. at Sierra Leone, Havana, Rio de Janeiro and Surinam, and with Foreign Powers on Slave Trade, 1831 (Class A & B), 38–40.

90. Cole and Macaulay to the Duke of Wellington. Sierra Leone, February 10, 1835. HCPP: Correspondence with British Coms. at Sierra Leone, Havana, Rio de Janeiro and Surinam on Slave Trade: 1835 (Class A), 49.

91. Report of the case of the Spanish brig "Formidable," Manuel Mateu, master. Sierra Leone, February 10, 1835. Ibid., 50.

92. Kilbee and Macleay to Canning. Havana, January 18, 1826. TNA: Foreign Office, 84/61.

93. W. Wilde to Lord Palmerston. St. Helena, March 4, 1850. And Abstract of the case of the brig "Aventuera." HCPP: Correspondence with British Coms. at Sierra Leone, Havana, Cape of Good Hope, Jamaica, Loanda, and Cape Verd Islands; Reports from British Vice-Admiralty Courts and Naval Officers on Slave Trade, 1850–51 (Class A), 139–40.

94. Lieutenant A. B. Hodgkinson to Captain Hastings. Prize Ventura, at sea, 70 16′ lat. South, 90 4′ long. East, February 2, 1850. Ibid., 246.

95. Thomas Butter to James Butter. HMS Sybille, Portsmouth, July 1, 1830. NMM: AGC/B/24.

96. Ibid.

97. Ouseley to Lord Palmerston. Rio de Janeiro, September 24, 1840. HCPP: Correspondence with Foreign Powers on Slave Trade, 1840 (Class B), 188.

98. Richardson to William Jeffery Lockett. HMS Maidstone, Sierra Leone, June 30, 1826. DRO: D8/B/F/66.

99. Graham E. Hammond to the Mixed Commission Judges. HMS Dublin, Rio de Janeiro, January 19, 1836. "Embarcação: Orion. 1834–35." AHI: Coleções Especiais. 53. Comissões Mistas (Tráfico de Negros). Brasil-Grã Bretanha. Lata 25, Maço 1, Pasta 1.

100. Statement by Mr. James Kittle, Surgeon of Her Majesty's ship "Cleopatra," September 21, 1844. HCPP: Correspondence with the British Commissioners at Sierra Leone, Havana, Rio de Janeiro, Surinam, Cape of Good Hope, Jamaica, Loanda, and Boa Vista, relating to the Slave Trade. January to December 1844 (Class A), 326.

101. Ibid., 326–27.

102. Ibid. Kittle's previous experience dealing with the spread of dysentery was key to his actions in this case. In fact, he was keen to remark that such an arrangement "made to prevent, if possible, the spreading of the disease on board, I deemed absolutely necessary, having seen the mischievous consequences of the infectious nature of dysentery on board Her Majesty's ship Andromache, when we lost 30 men"; ibid., 327.

103. Mr. [Hy] Piers' (Assistant Surgeon) Statement relative to the occurrences on board the prize "Progresso," June 1, 1844, HCPP: Correspondence with the British Commissioners at Sierra Leone, Havana, Rio de Janeiro, Surinam, Cape of Good Hope, Jamaica, Loanda, and Boa Vista, relating to the Slave Trade. January to December 1844 (Class A), 327–29.

104. Ibid., 328.

105. Ibid., 329.

106. Commander H. B. Young to Commodore Jones. HMS Hydra, off Quitta, March 7, 1845. HCPP: Correspondence with British Coms. at Sierra Leone, Havana, Cape of Good Hope, Jamaica, Loanda, and Cape Verd Islands; Reports from British Vice-Admiralty Courts and Naval Officers on Slave Trade: 1845 (Class A), 63–64.

107. For the Maria da Gloria see Fowell Buxton, The African Slave Trade, 178–80; and Harrison Rankin, The White Man's Grave, 2: 96–99. On the Arrogante, see Barcia, "White Cannibals, Enslaved Africans."

108. Bryson, Report on the Climate and Principal Diseases, 257.

109. Beveridge to Commander R. B. Crawford. [Simon's Bay], June 16, 1845. HCPP: Correspondence with British Coms. at Sierra Leone, Havana, Cape of Good Hope, Jamaica, Loanda, and Cape Verd Islands; Reports from British Vice-Admiralty Courts and Naval Officers on Slave Trade: 1845 (Class A), 126.

110. Donford to the Secretary of the Admiralty. Sierra Leone, May 16, 1845. HCPP: Correspondence with British Coms. at Sierra Leone, Havana, Cape of Good Hope, Jamaica, Loanda, and Cape Verd Islands; Reports from British Vice-Admiralty Courts and Naval Officers on Slave Trade: 1846 (Class A), 42–43.

111. Hill, Fifty-Days on Board a Slave Vessel, 79–80.

112. Mr. [Hy] Piers' (Assistant Surgeon) Statement relative to the occurrences on board the prize "Progresso," June 1, 1844, 329.

113. Bryson, *Report on the Climate and Principal Diseases,* 225–26.

114. Captor's declaration. HCPP: Correspondence with British Coms. at Sierra Leone, Havana, Cape of Good Hope, Jamaica, Loanda, and Cape Verd Islands; Reports from British Vice-Admiralty Courts and Naval Officers on Slave Trade: 1845 (Class A), 580.

115. Report of the case of the Esperanza. Sierra Leone, March 17, 1845; and Report of the case of the Bella Angela. Cape Town, August 14, 1844. Ibid., 197–98 and 201.

116. Statement of Mr. Henry Louey, Assistant-Surgeon of the HMS Vestal. HCPP: Select Committee on Slave Trade Treaties, Report, Proceedings, Minutes of Evidence, Appendix, Index (1852–53), 188. Sarsaparilla was an important item of trade in the Atlantic during the eighteenth and nineteenth centuries, often used to treat venereal diseases. See, for example, Burnard and Follett, "Caribbean Slavery, British Abolition"; and Gänger, "World Trade in Medicinal Plants."

117. Hill, *Fifty-Days on Board a Slave Vessel,* 110–11.

118. Ibid., 85.

119. Boyle, *A Practical Medico-Historical Account,* 382.

120. Alfred S. Pratt to Lieutenant C. H. Simpson. HMS Pluto, [at sea], November 30, 1859. HCPP: Correspondence with British Coms. at Sierra Leone, Havana, Cape of Good Hope and Loanda; Reports from British Naval Forces on Slave Trade: April 1859–March 1860 (Class A), 154.

121. Ibid.

122. Graham E. Hammond to the Mixed Commission Judges. HMS Dublin, Rio de Janeiro, January 19, 1836. "Embarcação: Orion. 1834–35." AHI: Coleções Especiais. 53. Comissões Mistas (Tráfico de Negros). Brasil–Grã Bretanha. Lata 25, Maço 1, Pasta 1.

123. De Monléon to the Baron de Mackau. Brig La Zebre, Sierra Leone, February 19, 1845. ANOM: Généralités, 166/1341.

124. Ibid.

Chapter 4. "Such an Asylum of Wretchedness"

1. The first slave vessel to be taken to Saint Helena was the *Julia,* which arrived with five African slaves on board in mid-December 1840. Pearson, *Distant Freedom,* 22–25.

2. Ibid., 107; "An Act for the Suppression of the Slave Trade." August 24, 1839 in *Anno Regni Vitoriæ Britanniarum Reginæ* (London: George Eyre and Andrew Spottiswoode, 1839), 741–4. See also "Lord Palmerston and the Portuguese Slave-Trade," *The Spectator,* November 9, 1839, 12.

3. As a matter of fact, McHenry threatened to resign his new post only five days after being appointed. George McHenry to Colonial Secretary William H. Seal, [Lemon Valley], December 25, 1840. SHGA: Colonial Secretary's In Letters 6, Vol. 2 (1840).

4. McHenry, "An Account of the Liberated African Establishment," 6: 253.

5. Edward Gulliver to William Henry Seale. St. Helena Marine Office, December 17, 1840. SHGA: Colonial Secretary's In Letters 7, Vol. 1 (1840).

6. Ibid.

7. Ibid.

8. McHenry to Captain Alexander. Lemon Valley, March 4, 1841. SHGA: Colonial Secretary's In Letters 7, Vol. 2 (1840–41); McHenry to John Young, Collector of Customs. Lemon Valley, April 24, 1841. SHGA: Colonial Secretary's In Letters 8 (1840–41).

9. McHenry, "An Account of the Liberated African Establishment," 6: 262.

10. Martinez, *Slave Trade,* 5–7. There were some exceptions, notably the temporary Key West depot established by the U.S. Home Squadron in early 1860. See Fett, *Recaptured Africans,* 70–72.

11. Pearson, *Distant Freedom,* 22–23.

12. Fyfe, *A History of Sierra Leone,* 1: 139, 160, 172.

13. Bethell, *The Abolition of the Brazilian Slave Trade,* 143–44. For some recent approaches to public health in nineteenth-century Rio de Janeiro see Franco, "O privilégio da caridade"; and Pimenta and Delamarque, "O estado da Misericórdia."

14. Nelson, "Slavery, Race, and Conspiracy."

15. These were not the only reception centers set up during the period. The French had similar depots in various parts of the Atlantic and Indian oceans— notably in the island of Gorée since the late 1820s—and the Americans established a similar type of facility in Key West in 1860 to deal with a number of Africans taken from slave ships seized by the U.S. Navy. See Daget, *La répression de la traite des Noirs,* 380. Fett, *Recaptured Africans,* esp. chapter 3; and Lawrence C. Jennings, "French Reaction to the 'Disguised British Slave Trade.' "

16. Bethell, "The Mixed Commission," 79. See also Nelson, "Liberated Africans in the Atlantic World"; and Scanlan, *Freedom's Debtors.* During this period there was also a Vice-Admiralty Court in Mauritius. See *Decisions of the Supreme Court.*

17. The abolitionist work of the Royal Navy and the courts of Mixed Commission and Vice-Admiralty was repeatedly questioned in London during this period, leading to a number of inquiries in the press and in Parliament.

18. The declaration was signed by Austria, France, Great Britain, Portugal, Prussia, Russia, Spain, and Sweden. Declaration of the Powers relative to the Universal Abolition of the Slave Trade, signed at Vienna, on February 8, 1815. Hertslet, *The Map of Europe by Treaty*, 1: 60–61.

19. The United States eventually signed a right-of-search bilateral agreement with Britain in 1862.

20. Smith, *The Lagos Consulate*.

21. For the *Isabel* see George MacDonald to Palmerston. Sierra Leone, July 7, 1851. TNA: Foreign Office, 84/831; and MacDonald to the Earl Granville. Sierra Leone, January 15, 1852. TNA: Foreign Office, 84/869; For the *Constancia* see "Return of slavers captured by H. M. Cruizers on the West Coast of Africa between 1st July and 31st Dec/60." TNA: Foreign Office 84/1150.

22. Eltis, *Economic Growth*, 131, 144.

23. They also used the services of amanuenses, interpreters, surgeons, and other petty officers.

24. Fifty cases were brought before the Havana Mixed Commission court and forty-four before the one in Rio de Janeiro.

25. Thomas Cole to J. Smart. Liberated Africa Department, August 23, 1828. SLPA: Liberated African Department; Letter book [19 August 1828–24 May 1830]. The best study to date on this second Middle Passage is Adderley, *"New Negroes from Africa."*

26. Figanière to [the Count of Palmilla]. Sierra Leone, August 14, 1821. ANTT: Documentos de Negócios Estrangeiros. Comissões Mistas. Caixa 224. Sierra Leone Papers.

27. Altavilla to Silvestre Pinheiro de Acevedo. Sierra Leone, August 9, 1821. ANTT: Documentos de Negócios Estrangeiros. Comissões Mistas. Caixa 224. Sierra Leone Papers.

28. Lefer Robaud to Ministro de Estado y del Despacho. Sierra Leone, November 30, 1819. AHN: Estado 8030, no. 34. The Dutch Mixed Commission arbitrator Mr. Bounurre was also forced to leave from Sierra Leone soon after his arrival for the same reasons. Gregory and Fitzgerald to Lord Castlereagh. Sierra Leone, April 4, 1821. TNA: Foreign Office 84/11.

29. Gregory's premonition was contained in a letter in which he begged George Canning to allow fellow judge Daniel Hamilton to return to England as soon as possible to save his life. In a twist of fate, only two months later, it was Hamilton who had to write to Canning informing of Gregory's death. Hamilton himself succumbed to the fevers too in 1826, as did Gregory's replacement, John Tasker Williams. Gregory to Canning. Sierra Leone, November 13, 1824; and Hamilton to Canning. Sierra Leone, January 15, 1825. TNA: Foreign Office 84/28.

30. Beginning in the late 1840s the arrival of various diseases, especially the yellow fever, combined with the poor hygienic conditions within the city, turned Rio de Janeiro into another propitious environment for the spread of disease. Candler and Burgess, *Narrative of a Recent Visit to Brazil,* 20.

31. Jameson, *Letters from the Havana,* 59.

32. Copy of a letter from Mr Deliège, lawyer, to His Excellence the Count Dessoble, Ministry of Foreign Affairs. Paris, June 20, 1819. ANOM: Sèries Géographiques, Amérique 16.

33. Abbot, *Letters written in the Interior of Cuba,* 244.

34. Ibid., 245.

35. A typical visit of this kind was that of Thomas Nelson to the *Dois de Fevereiro,* discussed in the Introduction of this book. These visits were carried out elsewhere in similar fashion. See, for example, Anderson, "Recaptives," 145.

36. Boyle, *A Practical, Medico-Historical Account,* 237.

37. Harrison Rankin, *The White Man's Grave,* 1: 106.

38. Cole to Ricketts. Liberated African Department, Freetown, June 15, 1829. SLPA: Liberated African Department; Letter book [August 19, 1828–May 24, 1829].

39. Denham to Lumley. [Freetown], September 30, 1827. SLPA: Liberated African Department; Letter book [February 11, 1827–August 19, 1828].

40. Huntley, *Seven Years' Service,* 1: 31; Misevich, "On the Frontier of 'Freedom,' " 204–43; and Anderson, "Recaptives," 159–210.

41. Young to Middlemore. Custom House, St. Helena, June 11, 1840. SHGA: Colonial Secretary's In Letters 9 (1841–42).

42. Pearson, *Distant Freedom,* 154–200.

43. Mamigonian, *Africanos Livres,* 90–95, 123–25, 130–31, 148–49, 253–56, 285–88, 304–6, 340–49, 360–66, 395–97. See also Jean, "A Storehouse of Prisoners"; and Nelson, "Apprentices of Freedom."

44. The Registry of Deaths that occurred at the Depósito between 1824 and 1845 suggest that even those who were considered to be healthy were still likely to die soon after being landed of infectious diseases probably contracted during the Middle Passage. See "Negros emancipados cuyos cadáveres consta en la parroquia del Cerro que se le remitieron del depósito de Cimarrones." ANC: Real Consulado y Junta de Fomento 149/7383.

45. Anglo-Brazilian Mixed Commission Court. Session of January 13, 1837. ANRJ: Junta de Comércio 184/4.

46. Hamilton to Canning. Sierra Leone, October 12, 1826. TNA: Foreign Office 84/49.

47. Colonial Surgeon [Boyle] to Colonial Secretary [Reffell]. Collector's Office, May 24, 1826. TNA: Foreign Office 84/49. In 1826 William Ferguson proposed

the establishment of a permanent "floating lazaretto for the reception of the sick Liberated Africans at their arrival." Response of Dr. W. Ferguson to questionnaire sent by the Commissioners of Enquiry. Sierra Leone, April 24, 1826. Sierra Leone Commissions of Enquiry. Vol. 2, Appendixes B and C. TNA: Colonial Office, 267/92. TNA: Colonial Office 267/92.

48. Anderson, "Recaptives," 144.

49. Leonard, *Records of a Voyage to the Western Coast of Africa,* 68.

50. Harrison Rankin, *The White Man's Grave,* 1: 352.

51. Clarke, *Sierra Leone,* 72.

52. Ibid., 73.

53. Pearson, *Distant Freedom,* 20.

54. Ibid., 108.

55. McHenry, "An Account of the Liberated African Establishment," 6: 151–55.

56. McHenry to Young. Lemon Valley, April 10, 1842. SHGA: Colonial Secretary's In Letters 11 (1842).

57. McHenry to Lord Stanley [the Early of Derby]. St. Helena, April 13, 1843. SHGA: Colonial Secretary's In Letters 14 (1843).

58. For a detailed chronology and examination of the facilities and medical care provided at Lemon and Rupert's valleys, see Pearson, *Distant Freedom,* chapters 4 and 5.

59. Deposition of Sir Charles Hotham, May 17, 1849. Select Committee of House of Lords to consider best Means for Final Extinction of African Slave Trade, Report, Minutes of Evidence, Appendix, Index. 130.

60. Young to Pennell. Custom House, St. Helena, March 27, 1848. SHGA: Colonial Secretary's In Letters 27 (1848).

61. Young to Pennell. Custom House, St. Helena, April 3, 1848. SHGA: Colonial Secretary's In Letters 27 (1848).

62. George Rowlatt to Pennell. Liberated Africans Establishment, August 9, 1851. SHGA: Colonial Secretary's In Letters 32, vol. 1 (1851); and Rowlatt to G. W. Edwards. St. Helena, May 14, 1852. SHGA: Colonial Secretary's In Letters 33 (1852).

63. Lima, Sene, and Souza, "Em busca do Cais do Valongo," 300.

64. "Noticias Marítimas. Navíos a Carga, Fretar e Vender," *Jornal de Comércio, Folha Comercial e Política.* Rio de Janeiro, July 21, 1830, 4.

65. Ouseley to Palmerston. Rio de Janeiro, April 14, 1840. HCPP: Correspondence with Foreign Powers on Slave Trade, 1840 (Class B), 155. See also Mixed Commission Court Session of January 13, 1837. ANRJ: Junta de Comércio 184/4, fol. 193v.

66. Ouseley to Palmerston. Rio de Janeiro, September 24, 1840. HCPP: Correspondence with Foreign Powers on Slave Trade, 1840 (Class B), 155.

67. "Asseisseira." AHI: Coleções Especiais. Comissão Mista. Brasil—Grã Bretanha (Tráfico de negros). Lata 02, Maço 02, Pasta 01.

68. McKinlay, "Remarks on the Yellow Fever," 339–40.

69. During particular periods, as it happened during the cholera epidemic of 1833, a far-reaching forty-day quarantine system was imposed on all vessels entering the harbor. Turnbull, *Travels in the West,* 252. See also "Supreme Board of Health, Sitting Extraordinary of 19 November 1833," *Diario de la Habana,* December 1, 1833, 1; and Francisco Dionisio Vives to the Secretary of State and Government. Havana, August 9, 1831. AGI: Santo Domingo, 1304.

70. Fernández de Madrid, "Memoria sobre la disentería," 381–89. Cf. Childs, *The 1812 Aponte Rebellion in Cuba,* 53; and Graden, *Disease, Resistance, and Lies,* 51–52.

71. Vives to the Mixed Commissioners. Havana, July 10, 1829. TNA: Foreign Office 84/92.

72. Madden to Kennedy. Havana, December 31, 1837. TNA: Foreign Office 84/240.

73. Bryson, *Report on the Climate and Principal Diseases,* 57.

74. *Report of a Special Committee,* 34–35; and *An Account of the Mercantile Marine Fund under the Act 17 & 18 Vict. c. 104.* Ordered by the House of Commons to be printed, April 20, 1860, 42; Saunders, "Liberated Africans in Cape Colony." See also George Napier to John Russell. Government House, Cape of Good Hope, July 27, 1841. NASA-CT: Papers despatched to Secretary of State, London: General Despatches. 1841. GH-23/13-75.

75. Reffell to Rev. M. Renner Leopold. Hospital, Leicester Mountain, December 18, 1820; Reffell to Tom Taylor. Leicester Mountain, December 9, 1820; and Reffell to Rev. G. R. Alexander. [Freetown], [March] 7, 1821. SLPA: Liberated Africans Department; Letter Book 1 (1820–26).

76. The questionnaires sent by the Commission of Enquiry are all located at TNA: Colonial Office 267/92. For the results of the enquiry see HCPP: Coms. of Inquiry into State of Colony of Sierra Leone, Report (Part I.); and HCPP: Coms. of Inquiry into State of Colony of Sierra Leone: Report (Part II.-Gambia, Gold Coast).

77. Response of Dr. Barry to questionnaire sent by the Commissioners of Enquiry. Sierra Leone Commissions of Enquiry. Vol. 2, Appendixes B and C. TNA: Colonial Office 267/92.

78. Response of William Ferguson to questionnaire sent by the Commissioners of Enquiry. Sierra Leone, April 24, 1826. Sierra Leone Commissions of Enquiry. Vol. 2, Appendix B & C. TNA: Colonial Office 267/92.

79. Response of Dr. Stewart to questionnaire sent by the Commissioners of Enquiry. Freetown, November 4, 1826. Sierra Leone Commissions of Enquiry. Vol. 2, Appendixes B and C. TNA: Colonial Office 267/92.

80. Kissy had long been praised as a more desirable destination for the reception of sick Africans, due to its better infrastructure and location. See, for example, "Sierra Leone," *Morning Chronicle* (London), October 6, 1823, 3.

81. Thomas Cole to [?]. Sierra Leone, October 20, 1828. SLPA: Liberated African Department; Letterbook [August 19, 1828–May 24, 1830].

82. Cole to John Dougherty. Liberated African Department, September 12, 1829. SLPA: Liberated African Department; Letter book [August 19, 1828–May 24, 1830].

83. "Quarterly Report on the State of Health of the Liberated African Population. 31 March 1830." By the Surgeon of the Liberated African Department, Andrew Foulis. SLPA: Liberated African Miscellaneous Return Book [1826–34].

84. Cole to Dr. Coker. Liberated African Department, Freetown, April 23, 1830. SLPA: Liberated African Department; Letter book [August 19, 1828–May 24, 1830]. Africans who had survived smallpox were always preferred for work at the hospital attending the sick. J. B. Mather to Dr. Coker. Liberated African Department, April 24, 1830. SLPA: Liberated African Department. Letter book [August 19, 1828–May 24, 1830]; J. Campbell to C. Jones. [Freetown], March 11, 1834. SLPA: Liberated African Department; Letter book [1831–34]; and C. B. Jones to G. Cummings. [Kissy], May 20, 1840. SLPA: Liberated African Department; Letter book [1837–42].

85. Leonard, *Records of a Voyage to the Western Coast of Africa*, 66–67.

86. Harrison Rankin, *The White Man's Grave*, 1: 352.

87. Clarke, *Sierra Leone*, 6.

88. Ibid., 71.

89. Ibid.

90. Over the following decades a grouping of smaller hospitals continued to exist in Kissy. At least one of them eventually turned into the psychiatric hospital that still exists today. See, for example, "The Kissey Hospitals," *Sierra Leone Church Times*, June 18, 1884, 2.

91. The reception center and lazarettos located in Lemon Valley were also considered to be a hospital in the early part of the 1840s. "Extract from Doctor McHenry's Letter, dated 22nd May 1843." SHGA: Colonial Secretary's In Letters, 14 (1843). See also Pearson, *Distant Freedom*, 26.

92. Gray, *Journals of Two Visitations*, 83.

93. Pearson, *Distant Freedom*, 111.

94. Ibid., 112.

95. Ibid., 112–13; Streatford to Seale. Royal Engineers Office, St. Helena, January 13, 1844. SHGA: Colonial Secretary's In Letters 17 (1843–44); and Rowlatt to Pennell. Liberated African Establishment, August 9, 1851. SHGA: Colonial Secretary's In Letters 32, Vol. 1 (1851).

96. For the use of the *Volant* as a floating hospital ship in 1842 see Vowell, Solomon and McHenry to Seale. St. Helena, November 28, 1842. SHGA: Colonial Secretary's In Letters, 13 (1842–43).

97. At some point after the asylum was closed, mentally ill patients were treated in the capital Jamestown. Vowell to Pennell. St. Helena, April 1, 1847. SHGA: Colonial Secretary's In Letters 20, Vol. 2 (1847); and Vowell to [?]. St. Helena, May 4, 1849. SHGA: Colonial Secretary's In Letters 28, Vol. 2 (1849).

98. Mamigonian, *Africanos livres,* 171, 177, 182–86, 194–96, 203–7.

99. Other vessels, like the *Carioca,* were also used for similar purposes in the early part of the 1830s. Mixed Commission Court session of July 29, 1835. ANRJ: Junta de Comércio 184/4.

100. Mixed Commission Court session of January 13, 1837. ANRJ: Junta de Comércio, 184/4.

101. Walsh, *Notices of Brazil,* 392, 417.

102. Rodrigues, *De Costa a Costa,* 293.

103. Ibid., 173–74.

104. Wurdemann, *Notes on Cuba,* 228.

105. "Informe de Tomás Romay." Havana, May 20, 1817. ANC: Gobierno Superior Civil, 1676/83838.

106. Romay to the Captain General [Miguel Tacón]. Havana, November 28, 1834. TNA: Foreign Office 84/151.

107. Macleay and Schenley to Palmerston. Havana, December 31, 1835. TNA: Foreign Office 84/172. The vessel arrived with so many of the crew and slaves sick that Macleay and Schenley referred to the mortality on board as "shocking," a term they rarely used. Of the 210 embarked, only 120 were still alive, many of them just barely, upon arrival, and the ship captain and a number of sailors had also died in the Middle Passage.

108. Madden to Kennedy. Havana, December 31, 1837. TNA: Foreign Office 84/240; Kennedy and Dalrymple to Palmerston. Havana, June 25, 1839. TNA: Foreign Office 84/274; and Kennedy and Dalrymple to James Bandinel. Havana, January 25, 1841. TNA: Foreign Office 84/347.

109. Holman, *Travels in Madeira,* 347–48.

110. Ibid.

111. Laird and Oldfield, *Narrative of an Expedition into the Interior,* 391.

112. Daniell, *Sketches of the Medical Topography,* 145.

113. Cape Colony was perhaps the healthiest and best-equipped British settlement throughout the entire South Atlantic. Pearson, *Distant Freedom,* 84.

114. Ibid., 83–84.

115. Leonard, *Records of a Voyage to the Western Coast of Africa,* 141.

116. Poole, *Life, Scenery, and Customs,* 2: 137.

117. Burton, *Wanderings in West Africa,* 1: 156.

118. "Report of Her Majesty's Commissioner of Inquiry on the State of the British Settlements on the Gold Coast, at Sierra Leone, and the Gambia, with Observations on the Foreign Slave-Trading Factories along the Western Coast of Africa, in the Year 1841." Appendix no. 3. HCPP: Select Committee on West Coast of Africa, Report, Minutes of Evidence, Appendix, Index, 11.

119. The representative for public works to the Presidente of the Junta Protetora de Escravos. Luanda, November 3, 1855. AHNA: Código 9/C-4-10, fol. 13v.

120. *Quarenta e cinco dias,* 38.

121. Clarke, *Sierra Leone,* 72.

122. Ibid., 73.

123. Pearson, *Distant Freedom,* 2.

124. Ibid., 159–60.

125. Hewett, *European Settlements,* 74.

126. Pearson, *Distant Freedom,* 84.

127. *A Report of the Trial of Pedro Gibert, Bernardo de Soto, Francisco Ruiz, Nicola Costa, Antonio Ferrer, Manuel Boyga, Domingo de Guzman, Juan Antonio Portana, Manuel Castillo, Angel Garcia, Jose Velazquez, and Juan Montenegro, alias Jose Basilio de Castro, before the United States Circuit Court, on an Indictment Charging them with the Commission of an Act of Piracy, on board the Brig Mexican, of Salem* (Boston: Russell, Odiorne and Metcalf, 1834), 27–30.

128. William Winniett to Chard. HM Brigantine Viper. At Sea, May 2, 1838. OUWL: Thomas Fowell Buxton Papers. Sections A-B. Mss. British Empire s. 444 (27). See also Pearson, *Distant Freedom,* 84.

129. Daniell, *Sketches of the Medical Topography,* 145–46.

130. Ibid.

131. Lima et al., "Em busca do Cais do Valongo," 307.

132. Pereira, *À Flor da Terra,* 26.

133. *Quarenta e cinco dias,* 30. Coghe, "The Problem of Freedom," 480–81.

134. Miller, *Way of Death,* 391.

135. When Reverend Abiel Abbot visited the lazaretto in the late 1820s he commented that although a large building, it was by then being neglected, its doors open and the patients—whom he referred to as Negroes—able to wonder around. Abbot, *Letters written in the Interior of Cuba,* 123.

136. Barcia, "El cementerio de los Protestantes," 80–82.

137. Representación de Dn. Ciriaco de Arango. Cabildo of March 5, 1818. AO-HCH: Actas de Cabildo Trasuntadas, Book 94, f. 77.

138. Barcia, "El cementerio de los Protestantes," 81–82.

139. On the Cape of Good Hope, for example, recaptured Africans were often relocated to Natal. P. Maitland to W. E. Gladstone. Camp near Buffalo Poorts. Kafirland, August 21, 1846. NASA-CT: Papers Despatched to Secretary of State, London: General Despatches. Introduction of Liberated Africans into Natal. 1846. GH-23/16-137.

140. Response of Dr. John Shower to questionnaire sent by the Commissioners of Enquiry. Sierra Leone Commissions of Enquiry. Vol. 2, Appendix B & C. TNA: Colonial Office, 267/92. TNA: Colonial Office 267/92.

141. Ibid.

142. Response of Dr. Barry to questionnaire sent by the Commissioners of Enquiry. Sierra Leone Commissions of Enquiry. Vol. 2, Appendixes B & C. TNA: Colonial Office, 267/92. TNA: Colonial Office 267/92.

143. Ibid.

144. Nelson, *Remarks on the Slavery and the Slave Trade of the Brazil,* 49.

145. Ibid.

146. Ibid.

147. Ibid., 49–50.

148. Macleay to Lord Aberdeen. Havana, August 28, 1828. TNA: Foreign Office 84/81.

149. Romay to the Captain General. Havana, November 28, 1834. TNA: Foreign Office 84/151.

150. Sandoval and Pérez y Carrillo to the President of the Junta de Medicine and Surgery. Havana, November 27, 1834. TNA: Foreign Office 84/151.

151. Ibid.

152. Macleay to Lord Aberdeen. Havana, December 15, 1828. TNA: Foreign Office 84/81.

153. John Young to Governor Middlemore. Custom House, St. Helena, June 11, 1840. SHGA: Colonial Secretary's In Letters 9 (1841–42).

154. McHenry to Lord Stanley. St. Helena, April 13, 1843. SHGA: Colonial Secretary's In Letters 14 (1843).

155. McHenry, "An Account of the Liberated African Establishment," 5: 435.

156. John Roby to Commodore P. J. Douglas. Custom-House, Montego Bay, July 23, 1838. HCPP: 1839 (162) *Ship Snake: Returns relating to the Portuguese slave vessel captured by Her Majesty's ship Snake,* 4. The mortality in this case seems to have been extremely high too: of the 407 Africans embarked at Gallinas, only 266 seem to have survived.

157. Lindon Howard Evelyn to Lord Glenelg. Lucea, February 17, 1838. OUWL: Thomas Fowell Buxton Papers. Sections A-B. Mss. British Empire s. 444 (28). See also Barcia, "White Cannibals, Enslaved Africans."

158. Stewart to Viscount Dudley. London, September 11, 1827. HCPP: "Papers Relating to the Slave Trade." Session January 29–July 28, 1828, 26: 23.

159. Rawlins to Young. [Jamestown], June 9, 1848. SHGA: Colonial Secretary's In Letters 27, Vol. 1 (1848).

160. Henry Hartley to Pennell. Liberated African Establishment, June 6, 1860. SHGA: Colonial Secretary's In Letters 42, Vol. 1 (1860–62).

161. Gregory to Canning. Sierra Leone, January 7, 1824. TNA: Foreign Office, 84/28.

162. Ibid.

163. Ibid.

164. Resignation of Dr. Meckleham. June 1835. TNA: Foreign Office 84/170; Kennedy to Lord Palmerston. Havana, June 24, 1839. TNA: Foreign Office 84/274.

165. McHenry to [Colonial Secretary?]. [Lemon Valley], December 20, 1840. SHGA: Colonial Secretary's In Letters 7, Vol. 1 (1840); and McHenry to Seale. Lemon Valley, March 16, 1841. SHGA: Colonial Secretary's In Letters 7, Vol. 2 (1840–41).

166. "Medical Report on the General State of Health and Quarters of the Liberated Africans at Bathurst. River Gambia, 31st December 1833." By Andrew Foulis, Assistant Surgeon in Medical Charge of Liberated Africans, R.A.C. and James Donovan MD, Acting Colonial Surgeon. OUWL: Thomas Fowell Buxton Papers. Sections C-D. Mss. British Empire s. 444 (28).

167. Voyages: The Transatlantic Slave Trade Database, at: http://slavevoyages.org.

168. "Return showing the number of Births and Deaths of Liberated Africans as reported to the Office by the Managers of the several Districts." Liberated African Department, Sierra Leone, July 9, 1830. SLPA: Liberated African Department Miscellaneous Return Book, 1826–34.

169. Ibid.

170. "Emancipados que fallecieron en el Hospital de la Casa del Dep° de 1824 á 1843." ANC: Real Consulado y Junta de Comercio 149/7383.

171. Pearson, *Distant Freedom*, 160–61.

172. Manoel Maria Rodriguez Bastos to [Young]. St. Helena, April 29, 1848. SHGA: Colonial Secretary's In Letters 28, Vol. 1 (1848).

173. Pliny Earle, "An Examination of the Practice of Bloodletting in Mental Disorders," *The New York Journal of Medicine and the Collateral Sciences* (New York: Purple and Smith, 1854), 13: 424.

174. Abstract of the case of the Spanish schooner "Josefa" (alias Maracayera), Joseph Moyano, Master, 1822. TNA: Foreign Office 84/16.

175. Boyle, *A Practical Medico-Historical Account*, 157.

176. Clarke, *Sierra Leone*, 90.

177. Leonard, *Records of a Voyage to the Western Coast of Africa*, 74.
178. Boyle, *A Practical Medico-Historical Account*, 137–39.
179. Ibid., 142.
180. Bacon, *Wanderings on the Seas and Shores*, 146–47.
181. Ibid., 148. Bacon may not have been, as he suggested, the first to manufacture this drug on African soil. References to practitioners capable of making their own medicines by mixing different chemical ingredients in the period are not rare. For example, Jerónimo Usera y Alarcón, upon arriving in Fernando Po in the 1840s, told of two resident practitioners and missionaries he encountered there who were able to prepare medicines "with their own hands." Usera y Alarcón, *Memoria de la isla de Fernando Poo*, 28.
182. Clarke, *Sierra Leone*, 89.
183. McWilliam, *Medical History of the Expedition to the Niger*, 194–95.
184. Bryson, *Report on the Climate and Principal Diseases*, 64.
185. "Invoice of medicines, &c., for the Liberated African department at Sierra Leone. Supplied by the acting Apothecary General, 3rd June 1834," SLPA: Liberated African Department Miscellaneous Return Book 1829–34; and McHenry to Young. Lemon Valley, November 2, 1842. SHGA: Colonial Secretary's In Letters 13 (1842–43). For the successful use of silver nitrate and the comparatively limited effectiveness of copper sulfate to treat ophthalmia, see also "Observations on the treatment of slaves by W. R. Stevenson, assistant surgeon RN. September 8, 1834. TNA: Foreign Office, 131/1, Part 2.
186. Bryson, *Report on the Climate and Principal Diseases*, 64.
187. Bacon, *Wanderings on the Seas and Shores of Africa*, 144.
188. *Quarenta e cinco dias*, 38.
189. Nelson, *Remarks on the Slavery and Slave Trade of the Brazil*, 55; Manoel Maria Rodrigues Bastos to Young. St. Helena, April 29, 1848. SHGA: Colonial Secretary's In Letters 28, Vol. 1 (1848–49). See also Journal of Her Majesty's Sloop "Rapid." Mr. Edward Heath Surgeon. Between the 2nd of January 1846 and the 2nd January 1847. TNA: Admiralty, 101/116/4.
190. "Expediente relativo a la salud y conservación de los negros en la travesía de la costa de Africa a este puerto." ANC: Real Consulado y Junta de Fomento, 150/7409; and "Informe de Tomás Romay, fecha Habana Mayo 20 de 1817, a la Junta Central de Vacuna sobre aplicación de la misma." ANC: Gobierno Superior Civil, 1676/83838.
191. Acta no. 8. November 8, 1850. Actas de Emancipados, 1850–63. AHNA: Códice 980 (2-3-29).
192. Deposition of Valentín José Pereira and António José López Soeiro, with British judge George Jackson present. Actas de Emancipados, 1850–63. AHNA:

Códice 980 (2-3-29). Like the Mixed Commission Court of Luanda, Robert Clarke complained about the unavailability of vaccines, mostly due to the fact that the lymph was being "destroyed by the climate." Clarke, *Sierra Leone*, 85.

193. Coghe, "The Problem of Freedom," 487–88. Compulsory vaccination was also applied at various times on African slaves along the African coast and in some parts of the Americas, notably in Cuba.

194. Usera y Alarcón, *Memoria de la Isla de Fernando Poo*, 54.

Chapter 5. A Shared Struggle

1. *Gibraltar Chronicle and Commercial Intelligencer,* August 4, 1828, 2. For American immigration into Cuba after 1817 see Barcia, *The Great African Slave Revolt,* esp. chapter 2; and Chambers, *No God but Gain.*

2. *Gibraltar Chronicle and Commercial Intelligencer,* August 4, 1828, 2.

3. Ibid.

4. Governor George Don to George Murray. Gibraltar, September 15, 1828. GNA: General Don's Despatches, 1827–32.

5. This principle also applied to the circulation of disease, especially epidemic ones, throughout the Atlantic.

6. Waserman and Mayfield, "Nicolas Chervin's Yellow Fever Survey."

7. For a range of opinions on whether Yellow Fever was contagious or not, see William Barnwell to Chervin. Philadelphia, April 30, 1821; and Franklin Bache to Chervin. Philadelphia, May 23, 1821. HML-CPP: Nicholas Chervin Papers, MSS 2/141. See also Antonio María Pineda to Chervin. Santo Domingo, August 6, 1818; and Michel Rolland to Chervin. Santiago de Cuba, January 26, 1819. NLM: Nicholas Chervin Papers, series 2. MS.C.20. Box 1, folder 7 (1/7). Letters. Haiti and Santo Domingo, 1818–19.

8. Bartolomé de Segura to Chervin. [Santiago de Cuba], [n/d], 1819. NLM: Nicholas Chervin Papers, series 2. MS.C.20. Box 1, folder 7 (1/7). Letters. Haiti and Santo Domingo, 1818–19.

9. Joaquín José Navarro to Chervin. Santiago de Cuba, February 28, 1819. Ibid. Navarro made these conclusions public only a few years before Audouard put forward his theory that yellow fever appeared and developed in the holds of slave ships.

10. Ibid.

11. Turnbull, *Travels in the West,* 224. According to *Voyages,* between 1817 and 1867, there were at least 157 slave ships that ended their transatlantic voyages at Santiago de Cuba, disembarking just under forty thousand African slaves in and around its harbor. The actual numbers are likely to have been much higher,

as numerous voyages lack specific details about final destinations or the numbers of Africans disembarked alive.

12. Chervin, *Réponse au discours de M. Le Dr. Audouard;* and Chervin, *De L'origine locale et de la non-contagion de la Fièvre Jaune.*

13. Smith, *Ship of Death.* See also Pym, *Observations upon the Bulam Fever.*

14. William Pym to George Don. Principal Medical Officers Office. Gibraltar, December 16, 1828. GNA: Despatches from Gibraltar, 1828. See also "Memorandum by Sir William Pym on provisions for quarantine at Southampton, after the outbreak of yellow fever in the West Indies, 1853." TNA: Public Record Office, 30/29/23/15.

15. D'Arcy, "William Pym," 84–85. See also Pym, *Observations upon Bulam, Vomito-Negro, or Yellow Fever.*

16. Bryson, *Report on the Climate and Principal Diseases,* 54–56.

17. Voeks, *Sacred Leaves of Candomblé,* 7–8, 161; Carney and Rosomoff, *In the Shadow of Slavery,* 166–70.

18. Bashford and Hooker, "Introduction," 2.

19. Gómez, *The Experiential Caribbean,* 141.

20. Ibid., 59.

21. Hopkins, *The Greatest Killer,* 181–84; and Kotar and Gessler, *Smallpox,* 86–100.

22. Burgo and Dew, *Science and Empire in the Atlantic World;* Castle, *Lexicon Pharmaceuticum,* 63, 203.

23. One such example was the suggestion of using "ice and ice-water externally and internally" for the treatment of fevers made in 1845 by a reader to *The Times.* "The African Fever," *The Times,* October 20, 1845, 8.

24. Duncan, *Travels in Western Africa,* 2: 145.

25. Ibid.

26. William H. Hole, "Account of a voyage to the coast of Africa, 1838–1839. At Cape Mount, October 5, 1838." BL: Rare Books and Manuscripts. Osborn d501.

27. Smith, *Trade and Travels,* 165.

28. Ibid., 166.

29. Mollien, *Travels in the Interior of Africa,* 52. See also Thévenot, *Traité des maladies des Européens.*

30. Lander and Lander, *Journal of an Expedition,* 2: 227.

31. Church, *Sierra Leone of the Liberated Africans,* 34.

32. Response of William Ferguson to questionnaire sent by the Commissioners of Enquiry. Sierra Leone, April 24, 1826. Sierra Leone Commissions of Enquiry. Vol. 2, Appendixes B and C. TNA: Colonial Office, 267/92.

33. Response of Mr. Bell to questionnaire sent by the Commissioners of Enquiry. St. Mary's, Gambia, June 24, 1826. Ibid.

34. "Report upon the state of the Liberated African Hospital at Kissy, commencing 1st August and terminating 31st December 1830, with a few remarks upon the state of health on the Colony generally for the last year." By J. Boyle, Colonial Surgeon. SLPA: Liberated African Miscellaneous Return Book, 1826–34, f. 191.

35. Ibid.

36. Dixon to Lumley. [Freetown], September 28, 1827. SLPA: Liberated African Department Letter Book [February 11, 1827–August 19, 1828], f. 133. This Mr. Brown was almost certainly William Brown, a maroon resettled in the colony who had been attending the hospital since 1826.

37. J. A. Schelky, [Circular]. Freetown, March 2, 1824. SLPA: Liberated African Department Letter Book [1820–26].

38. Clarke, *Sierra Leone,* 103.

39. Easmon, "Sierra Leone Doctors."

40. Ibid., 82.

41. Poole, *Life, Scenery and Customs,* 2: 137.

42. Holman, *Travels in Madeira,* 206.

43. Ibid.

44. McHenry to John Young. Lemon Valley, April 8, 1842. SHGA: Colonial Secretary's In Letters, 11 (1842).

45. Ibid.

46. Adeloye, "Nigerian Pioneer Doctors." See also Patton, *Physicians, Colonial Racism, and Diaspora.*

47. Horton, *West African Countries and Peoples.*

48. McWilliam, *Medical History of the Expedition to the Niger,* 246–47.

49. Clarke, *Sierra Leone,* 86.

50. Joaquín José Navarro to Governor Pedro Alcántara Suárez de Urbina. Santiago de Cuba, October 27, 1811. ANC: Correspondencia de los Capitanes Generales, 92/10.

51. Graham, *Journal of a Voyage to Brazil,* 283.

52. Ibid., 52.

53. "Existing obligations to baptize the libertos within 2 years and to vaccinate them by those who had taken them." AHNA: Códices, November 8, 1850; and Denham to Lumley. [Freetown], September 28, 1827. SLPA: Liberated Africans Department Letter Book [February 11, 1827–August 19, 1828].

54. McWilliam, *Medical History of the Expedition to the Niger,* 93, 247.

55. Ibid., 247.

56. "Relatorio do serviço de saúde do brigue Villa Flor 1854–1862." AHM: Documentação Avulsa, Caixa 469, Brigue Conde de Vila Flor.

57. Thompson, *The Palm Land*, 174.

58. Ibid.

59. Daniell, "On the Kola-nut of tropical West Africa"; Daniell, "Katemfe"; and Daniell, "On the production of hydrocyanic acid."

60. Daniell, *Sketches of the Medical Topography*, 93.

61. Ibid.

62. Ibid., 111–12.

63. Ibid., 38, 51.

64. Ibid., 129.

65. See, for example, McLeod, *Madagascar and Its Peoples*.

66. McLeod, *Travels in Eastern Africa*, 2: 286.

67. Ibid., 2: 289.

68. Ibid. For an entire list of the plants and remedies observed and described by McLeod see ibid., 2: 286–304.

69. Valdez, *Six Years of a Traveller's Life*, 246–47.

70. Ibid., 293.

71. Ibid., 127. Some of these plants appear in a report and inventory of Angolan medicinal plants written by Álvaro de Carvalho e Matoso in 1784. I would like to thank Kalle Kanooja for pointing me out in the direction of this important text. For a discussion of its content see Simon, "A Luso-African Formulary."

72. Winterbottom, *An Account of the Native Africans*, 1: 76, 2: 45.

73. Ibid., 2: 46.

74. Ibid., 1: 252.

75. Ibid., 2: 3.

76. Smith, *Trade and Travels*, 168.

77. "Relatorio do serviço de saúde do brigue Vila Flor 1854–1862." AHM: Documentação Avulsa, Caixa 469, Brigue Conde de Vila Flor.

78. Tucker and Smith, *Narrative of an Expedition*, 389.

79. Duncan, *Travels in Western Africa*, 2: 122.

80. Ibid., 2: 133.

81. Ibid., 2: 272.

82. Winterbottom, *An Account of the Native Africans*, 2: 2–3.

83. Hawkins, *History of a Voyage to the Coast of Africa*, 134; and Carnes, *Journal of a Voyage from Boston to the West Coast of Africa*, 379.

84. Pearson, *Distant Freedom*, 195–96.

85. McHenry, "An Account of the Liberated African Establishment," 2: 440.

86. Ibid.

87. Ibid.
88. Ibid., 441.
89. Thomas, *Adventures and Observation,* 218–19. See also Clarke, "Short Notes on the Prevailing Diseases," 67; and Bryson, *Report on the Climate and Principal Diseases,* 259.
90. João da Matta Chapuzat to Gobernor of Sao Jozé de Bissau. Ilha de São Thiago, June 22, 1825. No. 108. AHU: Gobierno de Guiné. Livro 32. Livro de Registro da Correspondencia entrada en Bissau enviada do quartel annual em Vila da Praia na Ilha de S. Tiago; and "Relação dos objectos necessarios para o Hospital Militar da Praça de Guerra de S. Jᵉ. de Bissau. 10 March 1844. Jozé Antonio Serrão, Governador Interino." AHU: Gobierno de Guiné. Livro 34. Livro de Registro da Correspondencia do Gobierno da Provincia dirigido a diversas autoridades. 12 Janeiro 1844 a 25 Novembro 1845.
91. Joaquím Antonio de Mattos to Caetano Procopio de Valdez. Bissau, November 23, 1830. AHU: Guiné. Caixa 24, no. 32.
92. Carlos [Maess] to the Duque of Cadaval. Arsenal Real da Marinha, [Lisboa], May 12, 1830. AHU: Guiné. Caixa 24, no. 10.
93. Miller, *Way of Death,* 429–30. See also Walter, "A propósito de uma doença de Angola"; and Rodrigues, *De Costa a Costa,* 258–59.
94. Rodrigues Bastos to Young. St. Helena, April 29, 1848. SHGA: Colonial Secretary's In Letters, 28, Vol. 1 (1848–49).
95. Ibid.
96. Ibid. See also Rawlins to Young. Rupert's [Valley], February 21, 1849. SHGA: Colonial Secretary's In Letters, 28, Vol. 1 (1848–49).
97. Usera y Alarcón, *Memoria de la Isla de Fernando Poo,* 28.
98. Owen, *Narrative of Voyages,* 1: 296.
99. Ibid. According to Owen, the so-called Marrello pill was made by mixing Peruvian bark and rhubarb.
100. Ibid., 193.
101. Mayer, *Captain Canot,* 69, 96–7, 273.
102. Ibid., 96.
103. Response of Dr. James Young to questionnaire sent by the Commissioners of Enquiry. London, March 26, 1827. Sierra Leone Commissions of Enquiry. Vol. 2, Appendixes B and C. TNA: Colonial Office, 267/92.
104. Fett reached this conclusion while examining the cases of the Africans found aboard four slave ships originating from different African regions, which were captured by the U.S. Navy and taken to Key West in the final years of the transatlantic slave trade. Fett, *Recaptured Africans,* 149.
105. Voeks, *Sacred Leaves of Candomblé;* and Brown, *Santería Enthroned.* On the relationship between another religion of African origin in the Americas,

Obeah, and the treatment of disease see Murison, "Obeah and Its Others"; and McGhee, "Fever Dreams."

106. According to Voeks, "Several centuries of plant introductions, intentional and accidental, between tropical Africa and the Americas, created a common domesticated and disturbance flora in these distant regions. "The Ethnobotany of Brazil's African Diaspora," 396–97.

107. Carney and Rosomoff, *In the Shadow of Slavery,* 88–89.

108. Chakrabarti, *Medicine and Empire,* 7–8.

109. Sweet, *Recreating Africa,* 149.

110. Gómez, *The Experiential Caribbean,* 130–31.

111. Weaver, *Medical Revolutionaries,* 113–24.

112. Deposition of Pancho Peraza. Ingenio Unión, Guamutas. March 1844. ANC: Comisión Militar, 36/2.

113. José Leopoldo Yarini, [Untitled manuscript, c. 1839]. AHCJF: Unclassified.

114. Ibid.

115. Apparently Pedro Gangá and Jacobo Lucumí attempted to kill the rest of Després family using the same herbs days later, failing only because the other intended victims found the taste of the coffee unpleasant. Another case, probably related to the events that transpired at the Unión, took place in an adjacent paddock, where another African slave, Camilo Macua, was accused of trying to poison his master. Depositions of José Gangá, José Lucumí, José María Congo, Pancho Peraza, Canuto Criollo, and Camilo Macua. ANC: Comisión Militar, 36/1.

116. Reis, *Divining Slavery and Freedom,* 136–37.

117. Gardner, *Travels in the Interior of Brazil,* 39.

118. Koster, *Travels in Brazil,* 255–56, 497–98.

119. Ibid., 255.

120. Ibid. For the most comprehensive list of Brazilian medicinal plants in the first half of the nineteenth century see Von Spix and Von Martius, *Travels in Brazil in the Years 1817–1820.*

121. Rodrigues, *De Costa a Costa,* 278–79; Pimenta, "Sangrar, sarjar e aplicar sanguessugas"; Dantas, "Barbeiros-sangradores."

122. Ewbank, *Life in Brazil,* 282.

123. Ibid.

124. Ibid.

125. Fett, *Recaptured Africans,* 149.

126. Macleay and Mackenzie to Lord Palmerston. Havana, December 22, 1832. TNA: Foreign Office, 84/128.

127. Walsh, *Notices of Brazil,* 415.

128. Ibid., 415–16.
129. Ibid., 415.
130. Ibid., 414.
131. Livingstone, *Missionary Travels*, 649.
132. Pearson, *Distant Freedom*, 19.
133. Shreeve, *Sierra Leone*, 41.
134. Ibid., 42.
135. Clarke, *Sierra Leone*, 90.
136. Pearson, *Distant Freedom*, 195.

Closing Remarks

1. Macleay and Charles Mackenzie to Palmerston. Havana, December 22, 1832. TNA: Foreign Office, 84/128.
2. An Account of the Deaths of Slaves on board the "Negrito" Spanish Slave Vessel, between the 21st November and 14th December 1832. Ibid. For a register of the Africans brought to Havana from the *Negrito* see TNA: Foreign Office, 313/58. I would like to thank Henry Lovejoy for bringing this register to my attention.
3. Diener and Manthorne, *El Barón de Courcy*.
4. Schiebinger, *Secret Cures of Slaves*, 3.
5. Rodney, *How Europe Underdeveloped Africa*, 96.
6. Clarke, "Short Notes on the Prevailing Diseases," 76. Although Clarke was specifically referring to Sierra Leone in this article, "white man's grave" was habitually applied at the time to the entirety of West and West Central Africa.
7. Ibid., 62.

Bibliography

Archival Collections

ANGOLA

Arquivo Histórico Nacional de Angola, Luanda (AHNA)

BRAZIL

Arquivo Histórico de Itamaraty, Rio de Janeiro (AHI)
Arquivo Nacional do Rio de Janeiro, Rio de Janeiro (ANRJ)
Arquivo Público do Estado da Bahia, Bahia (APEB)

CUBA

Archivo de la Oficina del Historiador de la Ciudad, Havana (AOHCH)
Archivo Histórico Carlos J. Finlay (AHCJF)
Archivo Nacional del Cuba, Havana (ANC)

FRANCE

Archives Nationales d'Outremer, Aix-en-Provence (ANOM)

GIBRALTAR

Gibraltar National Archives (GNA)

PORTUGAL

Arquivo Histórico da Marinha, Lisbon (AHM)
Arquivo Histórico Ultramarino, Lisbon (AHU)
Arquivo Nacional da Torre do Tombo, Lisbon (ANTT)

SAINT HELENA

Saint Helena Government Archives, Jamestown (SHGA)

SÃO TOMÉ E PRÍNCIPE

Arquivo Histórico, São Tomé e Principe (AHSTP)

SIERRA LEONE

Sierra Leone Public Archives, Freetown (SLPA)

SOUTH AFRICA

National Archives of South Africa—Cape Town Archives Repository (NASA-CT)

SPAIN

Archivo General de Indias, Seville (AGI)
Archivo Histórico Nacional, Madrid (AHN)

UNITED KINGDOM

Cambridge University Manuscripts Collection (CUMC)
Derbyshire Records Office, Matlock (DRO)
National Archives, Kew (TNA)
National Library of Wales, Aberystwyth (NLW)
National Maritime Museum, Greenwich (NMM)
Oxford University Weston Library (OUWL)

UNITED STATES

Beinecke Library, Yale University (BL)
British Art Center, Yale University (BAC)
Historical Medical Library of the College of Physicians of Philadelphia (HML-CPP)
Huntington Library, San Marino, California (HL)
National Library of Medicine, Bethesda, Maryland (NLM)
Sterling Memorial Library, Yale University (SML)

Newspapers

Diario de la Habana, Cuba
The Friend: A Religious and Literary Journal, London
Gibraltar Chronicle and Commercial Intelligencer, Gibraltar
Illustrated London News
Jornal de Comércio, Folha Comercial e Política, Rio de Janeiro, Brazil
Memorias de la Real Sociedad Económica de la Habana, Cuba
Morning Chronicle, London
National Anti-Slavery Standard, Monrovia, Liberia
The Observer, London
Sierra Leone Church Times, Freetown, Sierra Leone
The Spectator, London
The Times, London

Printed Primary Sources

Abbot, Abiel. *Letters written in the Interior of Cuba between the Mountains of Ar-
    cana, to the East, and of Cusco, to the West, in the months of February, March,
    April, and May, 1828.* Boston: Bowles and Dearborn, 1829.
"An Act for the Suppression of the Slave Trade." August 24, 1839. In *Anno Regni
    Vitoriæ Britanniarum Reginæ.* London: George Eyre and Andrew Spottis-
    woode, 1839, 741–44.
Adams, John. *Remarks on the Country Extending from Cape Palmas to the River
    Congo, including Observations on the Manners and Customs of the Inhabit-
    ants.* London: G. and W. B. Whittaker, 1823.
———. *Appendix Containing an Account of the European Trade with the West Coast
    of Africa.* London: G. and W. E. Whittaker, 1823.
Alban Imbert, Jean-Baptiste. *Manual do fazendeiro ou tratado doméstico sobre a
    enfermidade dos negros generalizado às necessidades de todas as classes.* Rio
    de Janeiro: Typographia Nacional, 1839.
Allen, William, and T. R. H. Thomson. *A Narrative of the Expedition sent by Her
    Majesty's Government to the River Niger, in 1841.* 2 vols. London: Richard
    Bentley, 1848.
Audouard, Mathieu F. M. "Mémoire sur l'origine et les causes de la fièvre jaune,
    considérée comme étant principalement le résultat de l'infection des bâti-
    ments négriers, d'après les observations faites à Barcelone en 1821, et au Port-
    du-Passage, en 1823." *Revue Médicale Française et Étrangère* 3 (1824),
    360–408.

Bacon, David Francis. *Wanderings on the Seas and Shores of Africa.* New York: Joseph W. Harrison, 1843.

Barnard, F[rederick]. *A Three Years' Cruize in the Mozambique Channel, for the Suppression of the Slave Trade.* London: Richard Bentley, 1848.

[Bel]. "Mémoire sur l'épidémie de fièvre jaune qui a sévi sur l'île de Gorée, pendant le quatrième trimestre de l'anné 1859." *Revue Maritime et Coloniale* 1 (1861): 194–238.

Bouët-Willaumez, Eduard. *Commerce et Traite des Noirs aux Côtes Occidentales d'Afrique.* Paris: Imprimerie Nationale, 1848.

Boyle, James. *A Practical Medico-Historical Account of the Western Coast of Africa: Embracing a Topographical Description of its Shores, Rivers, and Settlements, with their Seasons and Comparative Healthiness; Together with the Causes, Symptoms, and Treatment, of the Fevers of Western Africa; and a Similar Account Respecting the other Diseases which Prevail There.* London: S. Highley, 1831.

Bridge, Horatio *The Journal of an African Cruiser,* ed. Nathaniel Hawthorne. Aberdeen: George Clark and Son, 1848.

Bryson, Alexander. *Report on the Climate and Principal Diseases of the African Station; Compiled from Documents in the Office of the Director-General of the Medical Department, and from other Sources, in compliance with the Directions of the Right Honorable The Lords Commissioners of the Admiralty.* London: William Clowes and Sons, 1847.

Burton, Richard Francis. *Wanderings in West Africa from Liverpool to Fernando Po.* 2 vols. London: Tinsley Brothers, 1863.

Candler, John, and Wilson Burgess. *Narrative of a Recent Visit to Brazil.* London: Edward Marsh, Friends' Book and Tract Depository, 1853.

Carnes, J[oshua]. *A Journal of a Voyage from Boston to the West Coast of Africa: with a Full Description of the Manner of Trading with the Natives of the Coast.* Boston: John P. Jewett and Co., 1852.

Carpenter, William Benjamin. *The Physiology of Temperance and Total Abstinence. Being an Examination of the Effects of the Excessive, Moderate, and Occasional use of Alcoholic Liquors on the Health of the Human System.* London, Henry G. Bohn, 1853.

Carvalho e Menezes, Joaquim Antonio de. *Demonstração geografica e politica do territorio portugués na Guiné inferior, que abrange o Reino de Angola, Benguella, e suas dependencias.* Rio de Janeiro: Typ. Classica de F. A. de Almeida, 1848.

Castle, Thomas. *Lexicon Pharmaceuticum, or a Pharmaceutical Dictionary, comprehending the Pharmacopeias of London, Edinburgh, and Dublin, with a*

Variety of other Useful Information relative to Medicine and Pharmacy. London: E. Cox and Son, 1828.

Chateausaulin, Honorato Bernard de. *El vademecum de los hacendados cubanos ó guía práctica para curar la mayor parte de las enfermedades.* Havana: Imprenta de Manuel Soler, 1854.

Chernoviz, Pierre-Louis-Napoléon. *Formulário ou guia médico.* 6th ed. Paris: Casa do Autor, 1841.

Chervin, Nicolas. *Réponse au discours de M. Le Dr. Audouard contre le rapport fait a l'Academie Royale de Médecine de Paris, le 15 Mai 1827, sur mes documents concernant la Fièvre Jaune.* Paris: Crapelet, 1827.

———. *De L'origine locale et de la non-contagion de la Fièvre Jaune qui a régné à Gibraltar en 1828.* Paris: L'Imprimerie Royale, 1832.

Church, Mary. *Sierra Leone or the Liberated Africans in a Series of Letters from a Young Lady to Her Sister, in 1833 and 34.* London: Longman and Co., 1835.

Clarke, Robert. *Sierra Leone. A Description of the Manners and Customs of the Liberated Africans; with Observations upon the Natural History of the Colony and a Notice of the Native Tribes.* London: James Ridgway, 1843.

———. "Short Notes on the Prevailing Diseases in the Colony of Sierra Leone, with a Return of the Sick Africans Sent to Hospital in Eleven Years, and Classified Medical Returns for the Years 1853–4." *Journal of the Statistical Society of London* 19, no. 1 (1856): 60–81.

Couling, Samuel. *History of the temperance movement in Great Britain and Ireland from the Earliest Date to the Present Time with Biographical Notices of Departed Temperance Worthies.* London: William Tweedie, 1862.

Daniell, William F. *Sketches of the Medical Topography and Native Diseases of the Gulf of Guinea, Western Africa.* London: Samuel Highley, 1849.

———. "Katemfe, or the miraculous fruit of Soudan." *Pharmaceutical Journal,* October 1854, 158–60.

———. "On the production of hydrocyanic acid from Bitter Cassava root." *Pharmaceutical Journal,* 2nd series, December 1864, 302–4.

———. "On the Kola-nut of tropical West Africa (the Guru-nut of Soudan)." *Pharmaceutical Journal,* 2nd series, March 1865, 450–57.

D'Arcy, Power. "William Pym." In *Dictionary of National Biography 47,* ed. Sidney Lee. London: Smith, Elder and Co., 1896.

Davies, Rev. William. *Extracts from the Journal of the Rev. William Davies, 1st, when A Missionary at Sierra Leone, Western Africa.* Llanidloes: Wesleyan Printing House, 1835.

Decisions of the Supreme Court, Vice-Admiralty Court and Bankruptcy Court of Mauritius. London: William Maxwell, 1861.

Duarte, José Rodrigues de Lima. *Ensaio sobre a hygiene da escravatura no Brasil.* Rio de Janeiro: Typographia Universal de Laemmert, 1849.

Duncan, John. *Travels in Western Africa, in 1845 and 1846, Comprising A Journey from Whydah, through the Kingdom of Dahomey, to Adofoodia, in the Interior.* 2 vols. London: Richard Bentley, 1847.

Earle, Pliny. "An Examination of the Practice of Bloodletting in Mental Disorders." *New York Journal of Medicine and the Collateral Sciences* 13 (1854): 9–126.

Ewbank, Thomas. *Life in Brazil; or a Journal of a Visit to the Land of the Cocoa and the Palm.* New York: Harper and Brothers, 1856.

[Fawkner, James]. *Narrative of Captain James Fawkner's Travels on the Coast of Benin, West Africa.* London: A. Schloss, 1837.

Fergusson, William. *Notes and Recollections of a Professional Life.* London: Longman, Brown, Green, and Longmans, 1846.

Fernández de Madrid, José. "Memoria sobre la disentería en general y en particular sobre la disentería de los barracones." *Memorias de la Real Sociedad Económica de la Habana* 11 (1817): 381–89.

Foote, Andrew H. *Africa and the American Flag.* New York: D. Appleton and Company, 1862.

Fowell Buxton, Thomas. *The African Slave Trade and its Remedy.* London: John Murray, 1840.

Freeman, Thomas Birch. *Journal of Various Visits to the Kingdoms of Ashanti, Aku, and Dahomi, in Western Africa.* London: John Mason, 1844.

Gardner, George. *Travels in the Interior of Brazil principally through the Northern Provinces, and the Gold and Diamond Districts, during the years 1836–1841.* London: Reeve, Benham, and Reeve, 1849.

Gilliland, Herbert. *Voyage to the Thousand Cares: Master's Mate Lawrence with the African Squadron, 1844–1846.* Annapolis, MD: Naval Institute Press, 2004.

Graham, Maria. *Journal of a Voyage to Brazil and Residence there during Part of the Years 1821, 1822, 1823.* London: Longman, Hurst, Rees, Orme, Brown, and Green, 1824.

Gray, Robert. *Journals of Two Visitations in 1848 and 1850.* [Cape of Good Hope, 1850].

Hall, James. "Abolition of the Slave Trade of Gallinas." In *Twenty-Eight Annual Report of the American Colonization Society,* 33–36. Washington, DC: C. Alexander, 1845.

Harrison Rankin, F. *The White Man's Grave: A Visit to Sierra Leone, in 1834.* 2 vols. London: Samuel Bentley, 1836.

Hautain, Charles. *The New Navy List.* London: Simpkin, Marshall and Co., 1843.

Hawkins, Joseph. *A History of a Voyage to the Coast of Africa and Travels into the Interior of that Country.* Philadelphia: S. C. Ustich and Co., 1797.

Hertslet, Edward. *The Map of Europe by Treaty; showing the various Political and Territorial Changes which have taken place since the General Peace of 1814.* 2 vols. London: Butterworths, 1875.

Hill, Pascoe Grenfell. *Fifty-Days on Board a Slave Vessel in the Mozambique Channel, in April and May 1843.* London: John Murray, 1844.

Holman, James. *Travels in Madeira, Sierra Leone, Teneriffe, St. Jago, Cape Coast, Fernando Po, Princes Island, etc., etc.* London: George Routledge, 1840.

Horton, James Africanus Beale. *West African Countries and Peoples, British and Native. With the Requirements Necessary for Establishing that Self Government Recommended by the Committee of the House of Commons, 1865; and a Vindication of the African Race.* London: W. J. Johnson, 1868.

Howe, Julia Ward. *A Trip to Cuba.* Boston: Ticknor and Fields, 1860.

Huntley, Henry. *Seven Years Service on the Slave Coast of Western Africa.* 2 vols. London: Thomas Cautley Newby, 1850.

Jameson, Robert. *Letters from the Havana, during the year 1820; containing an Account of the Present State of the Island of Cuba and Observations on the Slave Trade.* London: John Miller, 1821.

Koster, Henry. *Travels in Brazil.* London: Longman, Hurst, Rees, Orme, and Brown, 1816.

Laird, MacGregor, and R. A. K. Oldfield. *Narrative of an Expedition into the Interior of Africa by the River Niger, in the Steam-Vessels Quarra and Alburkah, in 1833, and 1834.* London: Richard Bentley, 1837.

Lander, Richard, and John Lander. *Journal of an Expedition to Explore the Course and Termination of the Niger: with a Narrative of a Voyage down that River to its Termination.* 2 vols. New York: J. and J. Harper, 1833.

Leonard, Peter. *Records of a Voyage to the Western Coast of Africa in His Majesty's Ship Dryad, and of the Service on that Station for the Suppression of the Slave Trade, in the Years 1830, 1831, and 1832.* Edinburgh: William Tait, 1833.

Livingstone, David. *Missionary Travels and Researches in South Africa.* London: John Murray, 1857.

Matson, Henry James. *Remarks on the Slave Trade and the African Squadron.* London: James Ridgway, 1848.

Mayer, Brantz. *Captain Canot, or Twenty Years of an African Slaver. Being an Account of his Career and Adventures on the Coast, in the Interior, on Shipboard, and in the West Indies.* New York; D. Appleton and Company, 1854.

McHenry, George. "An Account of the Liberated African Establishment at Saint Helena." *Simmonds's Colonial Magazine and Foreign Miscellany* 5.18 and 20, 6.22–24; 7.25–26.

McKinlay, William. "Remarks on the Yellow Fever which appeared of late years on the Coast of Brazil." *Monthly Journal of Medical Science* 6 (1852): 335–52.

McLeod, Lyons. *Travels in Eastern Africa; with a Narrative of a Residence in Mozambique.* 2 vols. London: Hurst and Blackett, 1860.

———. *Madagascar and Its Peoples.* London: Longman, Green, Longman, Roberts, and Green, 1865.

McWilliam, James Ormiston. *Medical History of the Expedition to the Niger during the Years 1841–2, comprising an Account of the Fever which led to its Abrupt Termination.* London: John Churchill, 1843.

Mollien, G[aspar Theodore]. *Travels in the Interior of Africa to the Sources of the Senegal and Gambia; Performed by Command of the French Government, in the Year 1818.* London: Henry Colburn and Co., 1820.

Napier Hewett, J. F. *European Settlements on the West Coast of Africa, with Remarks on the Slave-Trade and the Supply of Cotton.* London: Chapman and Hall, 1862.

Nelson, Thomas. *Remarks on the Slavery and Slave Trade of the Brazil.* London: J. Hatchard and Son, 1847.

O'Byrne, William Richard. *A Naval Biographical Dictionary.* London: John Murray, 1849.

Ouseley, W. M. Gore. *Notes on the Slave-Trade with Remarks on the Measures Adopted for its Suppression.* London: John Rodwell, 1850.

Owen, W. F. W. *Narrative of Voyages to Explore the Shores of Africa, Arabia, and Madagascar.* 2 vols. London: Richard Bentley, 1833.

Philalethes, Demoticus, and Ignacio Franchi Alfaro. *Yankee Travels through the island of Cuba.* New York: D. Appleton and Co., 1856.

Pinto de Azeredo, José. *Ensaios sobre algumas enfermidades d'Angola.* Lisbon: Regia Officina Typografica, 1799.

Poole, Thomas Eyre. *Life, Scenery, and Customs in Sierra Leone and the Gambia.* 2 vols. London: Richard Bentley, 1850.

Pym, William. *Observations upon the Bulam Fever, which has of Late Years Prevailed in the West Indies, on the Coast of America, At Gibraltar, Cadiz, and other parts of Spain: With a Collection of Facts Proving it to be a Highly Contagious Disease.* London: J. Callow, 1815.

———. *Observations upon Bulam, Vomito-Negro, or Yellow Fever, with a Review of "A Report upon the Diseases of the African Coast, by Sir William Burnett and Dr. Bryson," proving its highly Contagious Powers.* London: John Churchill, 1848.

Quarenta e cinco dias em Angola: apontamientos de viagem. Porto: Sebastião José Pereira, 1862.

Reece, Richard. *Medical Guide for Tropical Climates. Particularly the British Settlements in the East and West Indies, and the Coast of Africa.* London: Longman, Hurst, Rees, Ormes, and Brown, 1814.

Report of a Special Committee of the House of Assembly of the State of New York on the Present Quarantine Laws. Albany: Carroll and Cook, 1846.

Ricketts, Henry John. *Narrative of the Ashanti War; with a View of the Present State of the Colony of Sierra Leone.* London: Simkin and Marshall, 1831.

Shreeve, William Whitaker. *Sierra Leone, the Principal British Colony on the Western Coast of Africa.* London: Simmonds's and Co. "Colonial Magazine" Office, 1847.

Sigaud, Joseph François Xavier. *Du climat et des maladies du Brésil, ou statistique médicale de cet empire.* Paris: Fortin, Masson and Cia, 1844.

Smith, J. *Trade and Travels in the Gulph of Guinea, Western Africa, with An Account of the Manners, Habits, Customs, and Religion of the Inhabitants.* London: Simpkin, Marshall, and Co., 1851.

Thévenot, Jean Pierre Ferdinand. *Traité des maladies des Européens dans les pays chauds, et spécialement au Sénégal, ou, Essai statistique, médical et hygiénique: sur le sol, le climat et les maladies de cette partie de l'Afrique.* Paris: J.-B. Bailliére, 1840.

Thomas, Charles W. *Adventures and Observations on the West Coast of Africa and its Islands.* New York: Derby and Jackson, 1860.

Thompson, George. *The Palm Land; or, West Africa, Illustrated.* Cincinnati: Moore, Wilstach Keys and Co., 1859.

Trobriand, Dénis de. *Une aventure de Négrier.* Le Havre: Chez J. Morlent, 1836.

Tucker, James Kingston, and Christen Smith. *Narrative of an Expedition to Explore the River Zaire, usually called the Congo, in South Africa, in 1816.* London: John Murray, 1818.

Tudor, Henry. *Narrative of a Tour in North America; comprising Mexico, the Mines of Real del Monte, the United States, and the British Colonies: with an Excursion to the Island of Cuba.* 2 vols. London: James Duncan, 1834.

Turnbull, David. *Travels in the West: Cuba; with Notices of Porto Rico and the Slave Trade.* London: Longman, 1840.

Usera y Alarcón, Jerónimo M. *Memoria de la isla de Fernando Poo.* Madrid: Imprenta de D. Tomäs Aguado, 1848.

Valdez, Francisco Travassos. *Six Years of a Traveller's Life in Western Africa.* 2 vols. London: Hurst and Blackett, 1861.

Von Spix, John Baptist, and Carl Friedich Philipp Von Martius. *Travels in Brazil in the Years 1817–1820. Undertaken by Command of His Majesty the King of Bavaria.* 2 vols. London: Longman, Hurst, Rees, Orme, Brown, and Green, 1824.

Von Zütphen, C. H. *Tagebuch einer Reise von Bahia nach Afrika.* Düsseldorf: Schreiner, 1835.

Walsh, R[obert]. *Notices of Brazil in 1828 and 1829.* Boston: Richardson, Lord and Holbrook, Crocker and Brewster, and Carter, 1831.

Winterbottom, Thomas. *An Account of the Native Africans in the Neighbourhood of Sierra Leone; to Which is Added an Account of the Present State of Medicine Among Them.* 2 vols. London: C. Whittingham, 1803.

Wurdemann, F. *Notes on Cuba, containing an account of its discovery and early history; a description of the face of the country, its population, resources, and wealth; its institutions, and the manners and customs of its inhabitants, with directions to travellers visiting the island.* Boston: James Munroe, 1844.

Secondary Sources

Adderley, Rosanne Marion. *"New Negroes from Africa": Slave Trade Abolition and Free African Settlement in the Nineteenth-Century Caribbean.* Bloomington: Indiana University Press, 2006.

Adelola Adeloye. "Nigerian Pioneer Doctors and Early West African Politics." *Nigeria Magazine* 121 (1976): 2–24.

Africanos na Santa Casa de Porto Alegre: obitos dos escravos sepultados no cemiterio da Santa Casa (1850–1885). Porto Alegre: EST, 2007.

Akyempong, Emmanuel, Allan G. Hill, and Arthur Kleinman, eds. *The Culture of Mental Illness and Psychiatric Practice in Africa.* Bloomington: Indiana University Press, 2015.

Anderson, Richard P. "Recaptives: Community and Identity in Colonial Sierra Leone, 1808–1863." Ph.D. diss., Yale University, 2015.

Androutsos, Georges, Aristide Diamantis, and Lazaros Vladimiros. "Le 'Rob de Laffecteur': un célèbre remède antisyphilitique aux temps des charlatans." *Andrologie* 18, no. 2 (2008): 172–79.

Arden, Dauril, and Joseph C. Miller. "Out of Africa: The Slave Trade and the Transmission of Smallpox to Brazil, ca. 1560–ca. 1830." *Journal of Interdisciplinary History* 18, no. 2 (1987): 195–224.

Armitage, David. "Three Concepts of Atlantic History." In *The British Atlantic World, 1500–1800,* ed. David Armitage and Michael J. Braddick, 11–29. London: Palgrave Macmillan, 2002.

Bankole, Katherine. *Slavery and Medicine: Enslavement and Medical Practices in Antebellum Louisiana.* London: Routledge, 2016.

Barcia, Manuel. "El cementerio de los Protestantes de la Habana." *Boletín del Gabinete de Arqueología* 1, no. 1 (2001): 78–83.

———. *Seeds of Insurrection: Domination and Resistance on Western Cuban Plantations, 1808–1848.* Baton Rouge: Louisiana State University Press, 2008.

———. *The Great African Slave Revolt of 1825: Cuba and the Fight for Freedom in Matanzas.* Baton Rouge: Louisiana State University Press, 2012.

———. *West African Warfare in Bahia and Cuba: Soldier Slaves in the Atlantic World, 1807–1844.* Oxford: Oxford University Press, 2014.

———. "Fully Capable of Any Iniquity: The Atlantic Human Trafficking Network of the Zangroniz Family." *Americas* 73, no. 3 (2016): 303–24.

———. "White Cannibals, Enslaved Africans, and the Pitfalls of the British Colonial System in Jamaica at the Time of Abolition." Keynote address. One-day Interdisciplinary Conference "Bites Here and There: Literal and Metaphorical Cannibalism across Disciplines." University of Warwick, November 17, 2018.

Barcia, Manuel, and Effie Kesidou. "Innovation and Entrepreneurship as Strategies for Success among Cuban-based Firms in the Late Years of the Transatlantic Slave Trade." *Business History* 60, no. 4 (2018): 542–61.

Barcia, María del Carmen, ed. *Una sociedad distinta: espacios del comercio negrero en el occidente de Cuba (1836–1866).* Havana: Universidad de la Habana, 2018.

Barnes, David S. "Cargo 'Infection,' and the Logic of Quarantine in the Nineteenth Century." *Bulletin of the History of Medicine* 88, no. 1 (2014): 75–101.

Barros, Juanita de. " 'Setting Things Right': Medicine and Magic in British Guiana, 1803–38." *Slavery and Abolition* 25, no. 1 (2004): 28–50.

Barros, Juanita de, and Sean Stilwell, eds. *Public Health and the Imperial Project.* Trenton, NJ: Africa World, 2016.

Barry, Boubacar. *Senegambia and the Atlantic Slave Trade.* Cambridge: Cambridge University Press, 1998.

Bashford, Alison. *Imperial Hygiene: A Critical History of Colonialism, Nationalism, and Public Health.* Basingstoke: Palgrave Macmillan, 2004.

———, ed. *Quarantine: Local and Global Histories.* London: Palgrave, 2017.

———. "Maritime Quarantine: Linking Old World and New World Histories." In Bashford, *Quarantine,* 1–12.

Bashford, Alison, and Claire Hooker, "Introduction: Contagion, Modernity, and Postmodernity." In *Contagion: Historical and Cultural Studies,* ed. Alison Bashford and Claire Hooker, 1–14. London: Routledge, 2001.

Beldarraín Chaple, Enrique. "Las epidemias y su enfrentamiento en Cuba (1800–1860)." Ph.D. diss., University of Havana, 2010.

Bethell, Leslie. "The Mixed Commission for the Suppression of the Transatlantic Slave Trade in the Nineteenth Century." *Journal of African History* 7, no. 1 (1966): 79–93.

———. *The Abolition of the Brazilian Slave Trade.* Cambridge: Cambridge University Press, 1970.

Braithwaite, Roderick. "The Rio Nuñez Affair: New Perspectives on a Significant Event in Nineteenth Century Franco-British Colonial Rivalry." *Revue Française d'Histoire d'Outre-Mer* 83, no. 311 (1996): 25–45.

——. *Palmerston and Africa: Rio Nuñez Affair, Competition, Diplomacy, and Justice.* London: I. B. Tauris, 1996.

Brown, David H. *Santería Enthroned: Art, Ritual, and Innovation in an Afro-Cuban Religion.* Chicago: University of Chicago Press, 2003.

Brown, Robert T. "Fernando Po and the Anti-Sierra Leonean Campaign, 1826–1834." *International Journal of African Historical Studies* 6, no. 2 (1973): 249–64.

Brown, Vincent. *The Reaper's Garden: Death and Power in the World of Atlantic Slavery.* Cambridge: Harvard University Press, 2008.

Bulmus, Birsen. *Plague, Quarantines, and Geopolitics in the Ottoman Empire.* Edinburgh: Edinburgh University Press, 2012.

Burgo, James del, and Nicholas Dew, eds. *Science and Empire in the Atlantic World.* New York: Routledge, 2008.

Burnard, Trevor, and Richard Follett. "Caribbean Slavery, British Abolition, and the Cultural Politics of Venereal Disease in the Atlantic World." *Historical Journal* 55, no. 2 (2012): 427–51.

Burroughs, Robert. "The True Sailors of Western Africa: Kru Seafaring Identity in British Travellers' Accounts of the 1830s and 1840s." *Journal for Maritime Research* 11, no. 1 (2009): 51–67.

Candido, Mariana. *An African Slaving Port and the Atlantic World: Benguela and Its Hinterland.* Cambridge: Cambridge University Press, 2013.

Canney, Donald L. *Africa Squadron: The U.S. Navy and the Slave Trade, 1842–1861.* Dulles, VA: Potomac, 2006.

Carney, Judith A., and Richard Nicholas Rosomoff. *In the Shadow of Slavery: Africa's Botanical Legacy in the Atlantic World.* Berkeley: University of California Press, 2009.

Carvalho, Marcus J. M. de. *Liberdade: rotinas e ruptras do escravismo no Recife (1822–1850).* Recife: EdUFPE, 1998.

Chakrabarti, Pratik. *Medicine and Empire, 1600–1960.* London: Palgrave Macmillan, 2014.

Chalhoub, Sidney. "The Politics of Disease Control: Yellow Fever and Race in Nineteenth Century Rio de Janeiro." *Journal of Latin American Studies* 25, no. 3 (1993): 441–63.

Chambers, Stephen. *No God but Gain: The Untold History of Cuban Slavery, the Monroe Doctrine, and the Making of the United States.* London: Verso, 2015.

Childs, Matt D. *The 1812 Aponte Rebellion in Cuba and the Struggle against Atlantic Slavery.* Chapel Hill: University of North Carolina Press, 2006.

Coghe, Samuel. "The Problem of Freedom in a Mid Nineteenth-Century Atlantic Slave Society: The Liberated Africans of the Anglo-Portuguese Mixed Commission in Luanda (1844–1870)." *Slavery and Abolition* 33, no. 3 (2012): 479–500.

Cohn, Raymond L. "Deaths of Slaves in the Middle Passage." *Journal of Economic History* 45, no. 3 (1985): 685–92.

Cook, Noble David. *Born to Die: Disease and New World Conquest, 1492–1650.* Cambridge: Cambridge University Press, 2010.

Costa, Valéria Gomes. "O Recife nas rotas do Atlântico negro: Tráfico, escravidão e identidades no oitocentos." *Revista de História Comparada* 7, no. 1 (2013): 186–217.

Crawford, Dorothy H. *The Invisible Enemy: A Natural History of Viruses.* Oxford: Oxford University Press, 2002.

———. *Deadly Companions: How Microbes Shaped Our History.* Oxford: Oxford University Press, 2009.

Crawford, Matthew James. *The Andean Wonder Drug: Cinchona Bark and Imperial Science in the Spanish Atlantic, 1630–1800.* Pittsburgh: University of Pittsburgh Press, 2016.

Crosby, Alfred. *The Columbian Exchange: Biological and Cultural Consequences of 1492.* Westport, CT: Greenwood, 1972.

———. "Virgin Soil Epidemics as a Factor in the Aboriginal Depopulation in America." *William and Mary Quarterly* 33, no. 2 (1976): 289–99.

———. "Infectious Disease and the Demography of the Atlantic Peoples." *Journal of World History* 2, no. 2 (1991): 119–33.

Curran, Andrew S. *The Anatomy of Blackness: Science and Slavery in an Age of Enlightenment.* Baltimore: Johns Hopkins University Press, 2013.

Curtin, Philip D. "The White Man's Grave: Image and Reality, 1780–1850." *Journal of British Studies* 1, no. 1 (1961): 94–110.

———. *Disease and Empire: The Health of the European Troops in the Conquest of Africa.* Cambridge: Cambridge University Press, 1998.

———. *Death by Migration: Europe's Encounter with the Tropical World in the Nineteenth Century.* Cambridge: Cambridge University Press, 1999.

Daget, Serge. *Répertoire des expéditions négrières françaises à la traite illégale (1814–1850).* Nantes: Centre de recherche sur l'histoire du monde atlantique, 1988.

———. *La répression de la traite des Noirs au XIXe siècle: L'action des croisières françaises sur les côtes occidentales de l'Afrique, 1817–1850.* Paris: Karthala, 1997.

Dalleo, Peter D. "Africans in the Caribbean: A Preliminary Reassessment of Recaptives in the Bahamas, 1811–1860." *Journal of the Bahamas Historical Society* 6 (1984): 15–24.

Dantas, Rodrigo Aragão. "Barbeiros-sangradores: as transformações no ofício de sangrar no Rio de Janeiro (1844–1889)" In Pimenta and Gomes, *Escravidão, doenças e práticas de cura no Brasil*, 248–72.

Diener, Pablo, and Katherine Manthorne. *El Barón de Courcy: Ilustraciones de un viaje, 1831–1833*. Mexico City: Artes de Mexico, 2006.

Domingues da Silva, Daniel B. *The Atlantic Slave Trade from West Central Africa, 1780–1867*. Cambridge: Cambridge University Press, 2017.

Dorsey, Joseph C. *Slave Trade in the Age of Abolition: Puerto Rico, West Africa, and the Non-Hispanic Caribbean, 1815–1859*. Gainesville: University Press of Florida, 2003.

Easmon, M. C. F. "Sierra Leone Doctors." *Sierra Leone Studies* 6 (1956): 81–82.

Eltis, David. *Economic Growth and the End of the Transatlantic Slave Trade*. Cambridge: Cambridge University Press, 1989.

———. "Fluctuations in Mortality in the Last Half Century of the Transatlantic Slave Trade." *Social Science History* 13, no. 3 (1989): 315–40.

Engerman, Stanley, and David Eltis. "Fluctuations in Sex and Age Ratios in the Transatlantic Slave Trade, 1663–1864." *Economic History Review* 46, no. 2 (1993): 308–23.

Everill, Bronwen. *Abolition and Empire in Sierra Leone and Liberia*. Basingstoke: Palgrave Macmillan, 2013.

Ferreira, Roquinaldo. "The Suppression of the Slave Trade and Slave Departures from Angola, 1830s–1860s." In *Extending the Frontiers: Essays on the New Transatlantic Slave Trade Database*, ed. David Eltis and David Richardson, 313–34. New Haven: Yale University Press, 2008.

———. *Dos Sertões ao Atlântico: Tráfico Ilegal de Escravos e Comércio Lícito em Angola, 1830–1860*. Luanda: Kilombelombe, 2012.

———. "Measuring Short- and Long-Term Impacts of Abolitionism in the South Atlantic, 1807–1860s." In *Networks and Trans-cultural Exchange: Slave Trading in the South Atlantic, 1590–1867*, ed. David Richardson and Filipa Ribeiro da Silva, 221–38. Leiden: Brill, 2014.

———. *The Costs of Freedom: Central Africa in the Era of Abolition (c. 1820–1880)*. Forthcoming.

Fett, Sharla M. *Recaptured Africans: Surviving Slave Ships, Detention, and Dislocation in the Final Years of the Slave Trade*. Chapel Hill: University of North Carolina Press, 2016.

Fohlen, Claude. "Une expédition négrière nantaise sous la Restauration." In *Les entreprises et leurs réseaux: hommes, capitaux, techniques et pouvoirs, XIXe–XXe siècles: mélanges en l'honneur de François Caron*, ed. Michèle Merger and Dominique Barjot, 157–66. Paris: Presses Paris Sorbonne, 1998.

Franco, Renato. "O privilégio da caridade: comerciantes na Casa de Misericórdia do Rio de Janeiro (1750–1822)." In *Filantropos da Nação: sociedade, saúde e assistência no Brasil e em Portugal,* ed. Gisele Sanglard, Luiz Otávio Ferreira, Maria Martha de Luna Freire, Maria Renilda Nery Barreto and Tânia Salgado Pimenta, 23–38. Rio de Janeiro: Editora FGV, 2015.

Fyfe, Christopher. *A History of Sierra Leone.* 2 vols. London: Longmans, 1962.

Games, Alison. "Atlantic History and Interdisciplinary Approaches." *William and Mary Quarterly* 65, no. 1 (2008): 167–70.

Gänger, Stephanie. "World Trade in Medicinal Plants from Spanish America, 1717–1815." *Medical History* 59, no. 1 (2015): 44–62.

Garland, Charles, and Herbert Klein. "The Allotment of Space for Slaves aboard Eighteenth-Century British Slave Ships." *William and Mary Quarterly* 42, no. 2 (1985): 238–48.

Gavin, R. J. "Palmerston Policy towards East and West Africa, 1830–1865." Ph.D. diss., University of Cambridge, 1959.

Gómez, Pablo F. *The Experiential Caribbean: Creating Knowledge and Healing in the Early Modern Atlantic.* Chapel Hill: University of North Carolina Press, 2017.

Gordan III, John D. *This Practice against the Law: Cuban Slave Trade Cases in the Southern District of New York, 1839–1841.* Clark, NJ: Talbot, 2016.

Graden, Dale T. "Interpreters, Translators, and the Spoken Word in the Nineteenth-Century Transatlantic Slave Trade to Brazil and Cuba." *Ethnohistory* 58, no. 3 (2011): 393–419.

———. *Disease, Resistance, and Lies: The Demise of the Transatlantic Slave Trade to Brazil and Cuba.* Baton Rouge: Louisiana State University Press, 2014.

Grenouilleau, Olivier. *Quand les Européens découvraint L'Afrique intérieure.* Paris: Tallandier, 2017.

Guizelin, Gilberto da Silva. "A abolição do tráfico de escravos no Atlântico Sul: Portugal, o Brasil e a questão do contraband de africanos." *Almanak Guarulhos* 5 (2013): 123–44.

Haines, Robin, and Ralph Shlomowitz. "Explaining the Mortality Decline in the Eighteenth-century British Slave Trade." *Economic History Review* 53, no. 2 (2000): 262–83.

Hallett, Robin. *The Penetration of Africa: European Exploration in North and West Africa to 1815.* New York: Praeger, 1965.

Harris, John. "Yankee 'Blackbirding': The United States and the Illegal Transatlantic Slave Trade, 1850–1867." Ph.D. diss., Johns Hopkins University, 2017.

Harrison, Mark. "Quarantine, Pilgrimage, and Colonial Trade: India 1866–1900." *Indian Economic and Social History Review* 29, no. 2 (1992): 117–44.

Head, David. *Privateers of the Americas: Spanish American Privateering from the United States in the Early Republic.* Athens: University of Georgia Press, 2015.

Helfman, Tara. "The Court of Vice Admiralty at Sierra Leone and the Abolition of the West African Slave Trade." *Yale Law Journal* 115, no. 5 (2006): 1122–56.

Hogarth, Rana A. *Medicalizing Blackness: Making Racial Difference in the Atlantic World, 1780–1840.* Chapel Hill: University of North Carolina Press, 2017.

Hopkins, Donald R. *The Greatest Killer: Smallpox in History.* Chicago: University of Chicago Press, 1983.

Howarth, Stephen. *To Shining Sea: A History of the United States Navy, 1775–1998.* Norman: University of Oklahoma Press, 1999.

Huillery, Elise. "The Impact of European Settlement within French West Africa: Did Pre-colonial Prosperous Areas Fall Behind?" *Journal of African Economies* 20, no. 2 (2011): 263–311.

Huzzey, Richard. *Freedom Burning: Anti-Slavery and Empire in Victorian Britain.* Ithaca, NY: Cornell University Press, 2012.

Jean, Martine. "A Storehouse of Prisoners: Rio de Janeiro's Correction House (Casa de Correção) and the Birth of the Penitentiary in Brazil, 1830–1906." *Atlantic Studies* 14, no. 2 (2017): 216–42.

Jennings, Lawrence C. "French Reaction to the 'Disguised British Slave Trade': France and British African Emigration Projects, 1840–1864." *Cahiers d'Études Africaines* 18, nos. 69–70 (1978): 201–13.

Jensen, Nicklas T. "Safeguarding Slaves: Smallpox, Vaccination, and Government Health Policies among the Enslaved Population in the Danish West Indies, 1803–1848." *Bulletin of the History of Medicine* 83, no. 1 (2009): 95–124.

Jones, Howard. *To the Webster-Ashburton Treaty: A Study in Anglo-American Relations, 1783–1843.* Chapel Hill: University of North Carolina Press, 2009.

Jones, Wilbur Devereux. "The Influence of Slavery on the Webster-Ashburton Negotiations." *Journal of Southern History* 22, no. 1 (1956): 48–58.

Kelly, Kate. *Old World and New: Early Medical Care, 1700–1840.* New York: Facts on File, 2010.

Kelly, Kenneth G., and Elhadj Ibrahima Fall. "Employing Archaeology to (Dis)entangle the Nineteenth-century Illegal Slave Trade on the Rio Pongo, Guinea." *Atlantic Studies* 12, no. 3 (2015): 317–35.

Kiple, Kenneth. *The Caribbean Slave: A Biological History.* Cambridge: Cambridge University Press, 1985.

———. "Mortality Caused by Dehydration during the Middle Passage." *Social Science History* 13, no. 4 (1989): 421–37.

Kiple, Kenneth, and Virginia Kiple. "Deficiency Diseases in the Caribbean." *Journal of Interdisciplinary History* 11, no. 2 (1980): 197–215.

Klein, Herbert, Stanley L. Engerman, Robin Haines, and Ralph Shlomowitz. "Transoceanic Mortality: The Slave Trade in Comparative Perspective." *William and Mary Quarterly* 58, no. 1 (2001): 93–118.

Kodama, Kaori. "Dr. Audouard in Barcelona (1821) and the Repercussions of His Thesis on Yellow Fever in Brazil." *Revista Latinoamericana de Psicopatología Fundamental* 11, no. 4 (2008): 805–17.

———. "Antiescravismo e epidemia: 'O tráfico dos negros considerado como a causa da febre amarela,' de Mathieu François Maxime Audouard, e o Rio de Janeiro em 1850." *História, Ciências, Saúde-Manguinhos* 16, no. 2 (2009). Online at http://www.scielo.br/.

Kotar, S. L., and J. E. Gessler. *Smallpox: A History.* Jefferson, NC: McFarland, 2013.

Law, Robin. *Ouidah: The Social History of a West African Slaving "Port," 1727–1892.* Athens: Ohio University Press and James Currey, 2004.

Lima, Carlos A. M. "Como se Cuba não existisse: observações sobre Jaime Balmes, a escravidão e o tráfico de escravos (Espanha, década de 1840)." *História: Questões e Debates* 50 (2009): 239–71.

Lima, Tania Andrade, Glaucia Malerba Sene, and Marcos André Torres de Souza. "Em busca do Cais do Valongo, Rio de Janeiro, século XIX." *Anais do Museu Paulista* 24, no. 1 (2016): 299–391.

Linebaugh, Peter, and Marcus Rediker. *The Many-Headed Hydra: Sailors, Slaves, Commoners, and the Hidden History of the Revolutionary Atlantic.* London: Verso, 2000.

Lockhart, Jamie Bruce. *A Sailor in the Sahara: The Life and Travels in Africa of Hugh Clapperton, Commander RN.* London: I. B. Tauris, 2008.

LoGerfo, James. "Sir William Dolben and 'The Cause of Humanity': The Passage of the Slave Trade Regulation Act of 1788." *Eighteenth-Century Studies* 6, no. 4 (1973): 431–51.

Longhurst, Peta. "Quarantine Matters: Colonial Quarantine at North Head, Sydney, and Its Material and Ideological Ruins." *International Journal of Historical Archaeology* 20, no. 3 (2016): 589–600.

López Denis, Adrián. "Cuerpos y prácticas. El cólera en la Habana en 1833." M.A. diss., University of Havana, 2001.

Lynn, Martin. "Britain's West African Policy and the Island of Fernando Po, 1821–43." *Journal of Imperial and Commonwealth History* 18, no. 2 (1990): 191–207.

Mamigonian, Beatriz. *Africanos Livres: A Abolição do Tráfico de Escravos para o Brasil.* São Paulo: Companhia das Letras, 2017.

Marques, João Pedro, *The Sounds of Silence: Nineteenth-century Portugal and the Abolition of the Slave Trade*. New York: Berghahn, 2006.

Marques, Leonardo. *The United States and the Transatlantic Slave Trade to the Americas, 1776–1867*. New Haven: Yale University Press, 2016.

———. "The Contraband Slave Trade to Brazil and the Dynamics of US Participation 1831–1856." *Journal of Latin American Studies* 47, no. 4 (2015): 659–84.

Martinez, Jenny. *The Slave Trade and the Origins of International Human Rights Law*. Oxford: Oxford University Press, 2012.

Martínez-Fernández, Luis. "The Havana Anglo-Spanish Mixed Commission for the Suppression of the Slave Trade and Cuba's Emancipados." *Slavery and Abolition* 16, no. 2 (1995): 205–25.

Massinon, R. "L'enterprise du Rio-Nunez." *Académie Royale des Sciences d'Outre-Mer, Bulletin des Séances* (1965), part 2, 304–53.

Mattos, Débora Michels. "Do que eles padeciam . . .: Doenças e escravidão na Ilha de Santa Catarina (1850–1859)." In Pimenta and Gomes, *Escravidão, doenças e práticas de cura no Brasil*, 63–89.

Mattos, Hebe, and Martha Abreu. "Relatório Histórico-Antropológico sovre o Quilombo da Pedra do Sal: en torno do samba do santo e do porto." In *O fazer antropológico e o reconhecimento de direitos constitucionais. O caso das terras de quilombo no Estado do Rio de Janeiro,* ed. Eliane Cantarino O'Dwyer, 23–67 (Rio de Janeiro: e-Papers, 2012).

McGhee, J. Alexandra. "Fever Dreams: Obeah, Tropical Disease, and Cultural Contamination in Colonial Jamaica and the Metropole." *Atlantic Studies* 12, no. 2 (2015): 179–99.

Miller, Joseph C. *Way of Death: Merchant Capitalism and the Angolan Slave Trade, 1730–1830*. Madison: University of Wisconsin Press, 1988.

Misevich, Phillip R. "On the Frontier of 'Freedom': Abolition and Transformation of Atlantic Commerce in Southern Sierra Leone, 1790s to 1860s." Ph.D. diss., Emory University, 2009.

Mouser, Bruce. "The Baltimore/Pongo Connection: American Entrepreneurism, Colonial Expansionism, or African Opportunism?" *International Journal of African Historical Studies* 33, no. 2 (2000), 313–33.

———. "Continuing British Interest in Coastal Guinea-Conakry and Fuuta Jaloo Highlands (1750 to 1850)." *Cahiers d'Études Africaines* 43, no. 172 (2003): 761–90.

———. "A History of the Rio Pongo: Time for a New Appraisal?" *History in Africa* 37 (2010): 329–54.

Murison, Justine S. "Obeah and Its Others: Buffered Selves in the Era of Tropical Medicine." *Atlantic Studies* 12, no. 2 (2015): 144–59.

Murphy, Laura T. *Metaphor and the Slave Trade in West African Literature.* Athens: Ohio University Press, 2012.

Nelson, Jennifer L. "Liberated Africans in the Atlantic World: The Courts of Mixed Commission in Havana and Rio de Janeiro, 1819–1871." Ph.D. diss., University of Leeds, 2015.

———. "Apprentices of Freedom: Atlantic Histories of the Africanos Livres in Mid-Nineteenth Century Rio de Janeiro." *Itinerario* 39, no. 2 (2015): 349–69.

———. "Slavery, Race, and Conspiracy: The HMS *Romney* in Nineteenth-century Cuba." *Atlantic Studies* 14, no. 2 (2017): 174–95.

Nerín, Gustau. *Traficants d'ànimes: Els negrers espanyols a l'Àfrica.* Barcelona: Planeta, 2015.

Newson, Linda, and Susie Minchin. *From Capture to Sale: The Portuguese Slave Trade to Spanish South America in the Early Seventeenth Century.* Leiden: Brill, 2007.

Ortiz, Fernando. *Contrapunteo cubano del tabaco y del azúcar.* 1940; Caracas: Biblioteca Ayacucho, 1987.

Palmer, Steven. "From the Plantation to the Academy: Slavery and the Production of Cuban Medicine in the Nineteenth Century." In *Health and Medicine in the circum-Caribbean, 1800–1968,* ed. Juanita de Barros, Steven Palmer and David Wright, 53–75. New York: Routledge, 2009.

Parron, Tâmis. *A política da escravidão no Império do Brasil, 1826–1865.* Rio de Janeiro: Civilização Brasileira, 2011.

Patton, Adell. *Physicians, Colonial Racism, and Diaspora in West Africa.* Gainesville: University Press of Florida, 1996.

Paugh, Katherine. "Yaws, Syphilis, Sexuality, and the Circulation of Medical Knowledge in the British Caribbean and the Atlantic World." *Bulletin of the History of Medicine* 88, no. 2 (2014): 225–52.

———. *The Politics of Reproduction: Race, Medicine, and Fertility in the Age of Abolition.* Oxford: Oxford University Press, 2017.

Pearson, Andrew. *Distant Freedom: St Helena and the Abolition of the Slave Trade, 1840–1872.* Liverpool: Liverpool University Press, 2016.

Pereira, Júlio César Medeiros da Silva. *À Flor da Terra: o cemitério dos pretos novos no Rio de Janeiro.* Rio de Janeiro: Garamond, 2007.

Pérez Morales, Edgardo. "Tricks of the Slave Trade: Cuba and the Small-Scale Dynamics of the Spanish Transatlantic Trade in Human Beings." *New West Indian Guide* 91, nos. 1–2 (2017): 1–29.

Pimenta, Tânia Salgado. "Barbeiros, sangradores e curandeiros no Brasil (1808–28)." *História, Ciências, Saúde-Manguinhos* 2 (1998): 349–72.

——. "Entre sangradores e doutores: Práticas e formação médica na primeira metade do século XIX." *Cad. Cedes, Campinas* 23, no. 59 (2003): 91–102.

——. "Sangrar, sarjar e aplicar sanguessugas: sangradores no Rio de Janeiro da primera metade do Oitocentos." In Pimenta and Gomes, *Escravidão, doenças e práticas de cura no Brasil*, 229–47.

Pimenta, Tânia Salgado, and Flávio Gomes, eds. *Escravidão, doenças e práticas de cura no Brasil*. Rio de Janeiro: Outras Letras, 2016.

Pimenta, Tânia Salgado, and Elizabete Vianna Delamarque. "O estado da Misericórdia: assistência à saúde no Rio de Janeiro, século XIX." In *Filantropos da Naçao: sociedade, saúde e assistência no Brasil e em Portugal*, ed. Gisele Sanglard, Luiz Otávio Ferreira, Maria Martha de Luna Freire, Maria Renilda Nery Barreto and Tânia Salgado Pimenta, 39–54. Rio de Janeiro: Editora FGV, 2015.

Pratt, Mary Louise. *Imperial Eyes: Travel Writing and Transculturation*. London: Routledge, 1992.

Quella-Villéger, Alain. *René Caillié, l'Africain. Una vie d'explorateur, 1799–1838*. Aicirits, France: Aubéron, 2012.

Ramsey, Matthew. "Academic Medicine and Medical Industrialism: The Regulation of Secret Remedies in Nineteenth-Century France." In *French Medical Culture in the Nineteenth Century*, ed. Ann La Berge and Mordechai Feingold, 25–79. Amsterdam: Rodopi B. V, 1994.

Reis, João José. *Divining Slavery and Freedom: The Story of Domingos Sodré, an African Priest in Nineteenth-Century Brazil*. New York: Cambridge University Press, 2015.

Reperant, Leslie A., Giuseppe Cornaglia, and Albert D. M. E. Osterhaus. "The Importance of Understanding the Human-Animal Interface." In *One Health: The Human-Animal-Environment Interfaces in Emerging Infectious Diseases*, ed. John S. Mackenzie, Martyn Jeggo, Peter Daszak, and Juergen A. Richt, 49–81. Berlin: Springer, 2013.

Rodney, Walter. *How Europe Underdeveloped Africa*. Cape Town: Pambazuka, 2012.

Rodrigo y Alharilla, Martín, and Lizbeth J. Chaviano Pérez, eds. *Negreros y esclavos: Barcelona y la esclavitud Atlántica* (siglos XVI–XIX). Barcelona: Ikaria, 2017.

Rodrigues, Jaime. *De Costa a Costa: Escravos, marinheiros e intermediários do tráfico negreiro de Angola a o Rio de Janeiro (1780–1860)*. São Paulo: Companhia das Letras, 2005.

——. " 'In This Trade, No Places Are Held': Involvement of Portuguese Slave Traders in the Slave Trade between Africa and Brazil (1818–1828)." *História (São Paulo)* 36, no. 39 (2017): 1–18.

Ross, David. "The Career of Domingo Martinez in the Bight of Benin, 1833–64." *Journal of African History* 6, no. 1 (1965): 79–90.

Ryan, Maeve. " 'A Moral Millstone'?: British Humanitarian Governance and the Policy of Liberated African Apprenticeship, 1808–1848." *Slavery and Abolition* 37, no. 2 (2016): 399–422.

Sanneh, Lamin. *Abolitionists Abroad: American Blacks and the Making of Modern West Africa*. Cambridge: Harvard University Press, 1999.

Santana, Jacimara Souza, and Andreilza Oliveira dos Santos. "Sangradores Africanos na Bahia do Século XIX (1825–1828)." *Sankofa: Revista de História da África e de Estudos da Diáspora Africana* 3, no. 6 (2010): 45–63.

Saunders, Christopher. "Liberated Africans in Cape Colony in the First Half of the Nineteenth Century." *The International Journal of African Historical Studies* 18, no. 2 (1985): 223–39.

Savitt, Todd L. *Medicine and Slavery: The Diseases and Health Care of Blacks in Antebellum Virginia*. Urbana: University of Illinois Press, 1981.

Scanlan, Pedraic X. "The Rewards of Their Exertions: Prize Money and British Abolitionism in Sierra Leone, 1808–1823," *Past and Present* 225, no. 1 (2014): 113–42.

———. "The Colonial Rebirth of British Anti-Slavery: The Liberated African Villages of Sierra Leone, 1815–1824," *American Historical Review* 121, no. 4 (2016): 1085–1113.

———. *Freedom's Debtors: British Antislavery in Sierra Leone in the Age of Revolution*. New Haven: Yale University Press, 2017.

Schiebinger, Londa. *Secret Cures of Slaves: People, Plants, and Medicine in the Eighteenth-Century Atlantic World*. Stanford: Stanford University Press, 2017.

Senior, Emily. *The Caribbean and the Medical Imagination, 1764–1834: Slavery, Disease, and Colonial Modernity*. Cambridge: Cambridge University Press, 2018.

Shaikh, Farida. "Judicial Diplomacy: British Officials and the Mixed Commission Courts." In *Slavery, Diplomacy, and Empire: Britain and the Suppression of the Slave Trade, 1807–1975*, ed. Keith Hamilton and Patrick Salmon, 42–64. Brighton: Sussex Academic Press, 2009.

Sheridan, Richard. "The Guinea Surgeons on the Middle Passage: The Provision of Medical Services in the British Slave Trade." *International Journal of African Historical Studies* 14, no. 4 (1981): 601–25.

———. *Doctors and Slaves: A Medical and Demographic History of Slavery in the British West Indies, 1680–1834*. Cambridge: Cambridge University Press, 1985.

Silva, Ricardo Tadeu Caíres. "Memórias do tráfico illegal de escravos nas ações de liberdade, 1885–1888." *Afro-Ásia* 35 (2007): 37–82.

Simon, William J. "A Luso-African Formulary of the Late Eighteenth Century: Some Notes on Angolan Contributions to European Knowledge of Material Medica." *Pharmacy in History* 18, no. 3 (1976): 103–14.

Smith, Billy G. *Ship of Death: A Voyage That Changed the Atlantic World.* New Haven: Yale University Press, 2013.

Smith, Robert S. *The Lagos Consulate.* Berkeley: University of California Press, 1979.

Soumonni, Elisée. "Lacustrine Villages in South Benin as Refugees from the Slave Trade." In *Fighting the Slave Trade: West African Strategies,* ed. Sylviane Diouf, 3–14. Athens: Ohio University Press and James Currey, 2003.

Sparks, Randy J. *Where the Negroes Are Masters: An African Port in the Era of the Slave Trade.* Cambridge: Harvard University Press, 2014.

Steckel, Richard H., and Richard A. Jensen. "New Evidence on the Causes of Slave and Crew Mortality in the Atlantic Slave Trade." *Journal of Economic History* 46, no. 1 (1986): 57–77.

Sweet, James H. *Recreating Africa: Culture, Kingship, and Religion in the African-Portuguese World, 1441–1770.* Chapel Hill: University of North Carolina Press, 2003.

Temperley, Howard. *White Dreams, Black Africa: The Antislavery Expedition to the Niger.* New Haven: Yale University Press, 1991.

Thornton John K. *Africa and the Africans in the Making of the Atlantic World, 1400–1800.* Cambridge: Cambridge University Press, 1992.

———. *Warfare in Atlantic Africa, 1500–1800.* London: UCL Press, 1999.

Tilma Sauer and Raphael Scholl, eds. *The Philosophy of Historical Case Studies.* Basel: Springer, 2016, 265–84.

Tinnie, Dinizulu Gene. "The Slaving Brig *Henriqueta* and Her Evil Sisters: A Case Study in the 19th-Century Slave Trade to Brazil." *Journal of African American History* 93, no. 4 (2008): 509–31.

Tognotti, Eugenia. "Lessons from the History of Quarantine, from Plague to Influenza A." *Emerging Infectious Diseases* 19, no. 2 (2013): 254–59.

Tulodziecki, Dana. "From Zymes to Germs: Discarding the Realist/Anti-Realist Framework." In *The Philosophy of Historical Case-Studies,* ed. Tilman Sauer and Raphael Scholl, 265–84. New York: Springer, 2016.

Tyler-McGraw, Marie. *An African Republic: Black and White Virginians in the Making of Liberia.* Chapel Hill: University of North Carolina Press, 2007.

Van Norman, William C., Jr. "The Process of Cultural Change among Cuban Bozales during the Nineteenth Century." *The Americas* 62, no. 2 (2005): 177–207.

Vaughan, Megan. *Curing Their Ills: Colonial Power and African Illness.* Cambridge: Polity, 1991.

Viana Filho, Luis. *O negro na Bahia.* Rio de Janeiro: José Olympio, 1946.

Voeks, Robert A. *Sacred Leaves of Candomblé: African Magic, Medicine, and Religion in Brazil.* Austin: University of Texas Press, 1997.

———. "The Ethnobotany of Brazil's African Diaspora: The Role of Floristic Homogenization." In *African Ethnobotany in the Americas,* ed. Robert Voeks and John Rashford, 395–416. New York: Springer, 2013.

Walter, Jaime. "A propósito de uma doença de Angola de há mais de três séculos: doença do bicho ou maculo." *Boletim clínico e estatístico do Hospital do Ultramar* 7 (1957): 47–68.

Waserman, Manfred J., and Virginia Kay Mayfield. "Nicolas Chervin's Yellow Fever Survey, 1820–1822." *Journal of the History of Medicine and Allied Sciences* 26, no. 1 (1971): 40–51.

Watt, James. "The Health of Seamen in Anti-Slavery Squadrons." *Mariner's Mirror* 88, no. 1 (2002): 69–78.

Weaver, Karol K. *Medical Revolutionaries: The Enslaved Healers of Eighteenth-Century Saint Domingue.* Urbana: University of Illinois Press, 2006.

Weiner, Marli F., and Mazie Hough. *Sex, Sickness, and Slavery: Illness in the Antebellum South.* Urbana: University of Illinois Press, 2012.

Michael Zeuske. *Amistad: A Hidden Network of Slavers and Merchants.* Princeton: Markus Wiener, 2014.

———. "Cosmopólitas del Atlántico esclavista: los 'africanos' Daniel Botefeur y su esclavos de confianza Robin Botefeur en Cuba." *Almanack* 12 (2016): 129–55.

Index